# Wellness Tech Innovations in Health Monitoring

# Wellness Tech Innovations in Health Monitoring

Rafeal Mechlore

UNIEK ENTERPRISES

# Contents

# INDEX

**Chapter 1: Introduction**



**Chapter 2: Wearable Devices and Health Tracking**



**Chapter 3: Remote Patient Monitoring**



**Chapter 4: Smart Health Apps and Platforms**



**Chapter 5: Artificial Intelligence in Health Monitoring**

# *Chapter 1*

## Introduction

As of late, the crossing point of innovation and medical services has led to a groundbreaking flood of developments that are reshaping the scene of wellbeing observing. As social orders across the globe wrestle with the difficulties presented by a maturing populace, raising medical care costs, and the rising pervasiveness of ongoing sicknesses, there is a developing acknowledgment of the requirement for proactive and customized ways to deal with medical services. Because of these difficulties, the development of wellbeing tech has turned into a point of convergence, offering a range of instruments and arrangements intended to enable people in dealing with their wellbeing and prosperity.

Wellbeing tech, a general classification enveloping a different exhibit of advancements, has picked up speed as a powerful power driving change in medical care rehearses. From wearable gadgets to portable applications and high level sensors, these developments are not just giving people remarkable bits of knowledge into their wellbeing but at the same time are cultivating a shift towards preventive medical care. The customary model of medical services, portrayed by receptive intercessions and wordy consideration, is slowly giving way to a more all encompassing and consistent methodology worked with by health tech.

At the core of this change is the combination of state of the art innovation with wellbeing checking, making a collaboration that goes past simple information assortment. The joining of man-made consciousness (simulated intelligence), AI, and huge information investigation has pushed wellbeing tech into a domain where it can decipher complex wellbeing measurements, recognize designs, and convey significant experiences.

This blend of innovation and wellbeing is enabling people to play a more dynamic job in their prosperity, introducing a time of customized, information driven medical services.

One of the significant components driving the flood in wellbeing tech reception is the rising pervasiveness of wearable gadgets. These conservative, sensor-loaded contraptions play rose above their underlying part as wellness trackers and advanced into exhaustive wellbeing observing devices. Whether as smartwatches, wellness groups, or even brilliant dress, wearables are currently fit for checking a huge number of wellbeing boundaries, including pulse, rest designs, active work, and even feelings of anxiety. The ongoing information created by these gadgets empowers clients to acquire a nuanced comprehension of their wellbeing, encouraging a feeling of strengthening and informed independent direction.

At the same time, portable applications have arisen as basic allies to wearable gadgets, filling in as unified center points for wellbeing information and bits of knowledge. These applications work with consistent incorporation with wearables as well as give highlights, for example, customized wellbeing suggestions, objective following, and local area commitment. The collaboration among wearables and versatile applications makes a durable environment that changes wellbeing checking into an intelligent and client driven insight.

Notwithstanding wearables and portable applications, the approach of shrewd sensors and associated gadgets is extending the extent of health tech. These sensors, implanted in regular items or coordinated into the living climate, can possibly catch an extensive variety of wellbeing related information without the requirement for unequivocal client input. Brilliant home gadgets, for example, can screen factors like air quality, temperature, and even recognize falls, adding to a comprehensive comprehension of a singular's prosperity. The expansion of such sensor-based advances is obscuring the lines between conventional medical care settings and the ordinary spaces individuals occupy.

Significant to the extraordinary capability of wellbeing tech is the job of computerized reasoning and AI calculations. These cutting edge innovations, filled by immense measures of wellbeing information, have the ability to investigate complex examples, anticipate wellbeing results, and create customized suggestions. AI calculations can filter through huge datasets to distinguish unobtrusive connections, empowering early discovery of medical problems and fitting mediations in light of individual wellbeing profiles. As simulated intelligence keeps on developing, its reconciliation into wellbeing tech is ready to reform wellbeing checking by upgrading precision, prescient capacities, and the general viability of customized mediations.

The shift towards proactive wellbeing the executives worked with by health tech isn't just impacting people but at the same time is resounding across medical care frameworks and establishments.

The reception of distant patient checking (RPM) is picking up speed, permitting medical services suppliers to screen patients' important bodily functions and wellbeing measurements beyond customary clinical settings. This improves patient comfort as well as empowers early location of decaying medical issue, lessening the weight on medical care offices and bringing down generally medical services costs.

In addition, wellbeing tech is adding to the democratization of medical care by cultivating more prominent admittance to wellbeing data and assets. The openness of wellbeing related applications, wearables, and online stages rises above geological limits, giving people in remote or underserved regions with devices to screen and deal with their wellbeing. This democratization is especially critical with regards to preventive consideration, as people gain the means to proactively address wellbeing worries before they heighten, no matter what their area or financial status.

Regardless of the groundbreaking capability of wellbeing tech, its quick development isn't without difficulties and contemplations. Protection concerns encompassing the assortment and usage of individual wellbeing information pose a potential threat, provoking a basic assessment of information safety efforts and moral contemplations. Finding some kind of harmony between the advantages of customized wellbeing experiences and the security of individual protection is a squeezing worry that requires insightful administrative structures and straightforward correspondence from tech engineers.

Besides, the viability and precision of health tech advancements warrant progressing approval and refinement. While these advancements hold enormous commitment, guaranteeing their unwavering quality and exactness in different populaces and certifiable situations is pivotal for laying out trust among clients and medical care experts the same. Joint efforts between tech engineers, medical services suppliers, and administrative bodies are fundamental for set strong norms and guarantee that wellbeing tech meets the thorough necessities of the medical services scene.

As wellbeing tech keeps on advancing, its effect isn't restricted to individual wellbeing checking; it stretches out to general wellbeing drives and exploration tries. The collection of anonymized and totaled information from huge client bases sets out open doors for epidemiological examinations, infection reconnaissance, and the ID of wellbeing patterns at a populace level. Outfitting the force of wellbeing tech information on a more extensive scale can possibly illuminate general wellbeing strategies, shape preventive procedures, and add to the progression of clinical information.

## 1.1 Overview of the rapidly evolving landscape of wellness technology

The contemporary medical care scene is seeing a significant change filled by the fast combination of innovation into the domain of health. As the interest for more proactive and customized medical care arrangements develops, wellbeing innovation has arisen as a unique power, reshaping the manner in which people see and deal with their wellbeing. This developing scene includes a different cluster of advancements, going from wearable gadgets and portable applications to cutting edge sensors and man-made consciousness (simulated intelligence) calculations. The intermingling of these innovations is driving a change in perspective towards preventive medical care, engaging people with devices to screen, comprehend, and improve their prosperity.

At the very front of this advancement are wearable gadgets, which play rose above their underlying part as wellness trackers to become refined wellbeing checking devices. These minimal contraptions, frequently as smartwatches, wellness groups, or even brilliant apparel, are furnished with a variety of sensors equipped for following different wellbeing measurements. From checking pulse and rest examples to evaluating actual work and feelings of anxiety, wearables furnish clients with ongoing information, offering experiences into their general wellbeing. The omnipresence of these gadgets has changed wellbeing observing from a periodic movement to a constant, ordinary experience, cultivating a feeling of mindfulness and commitment to one's own wellbeing.

Supplementing wearables are portable applications that act as focal centers for wellbeing information accumulation, examination, and understanding. These applications consistently incorporate with wearables, making a brought together biological system that merges wellbeing related data. Past simple information stockpiling, these applications give highlights, for example, customized wellbeing suggestions, objective following, and social network. By furnishing clients with significant bits of knowledge and cultivating a feeling of local area, versatile applications upgrade the client experience and add to the more extensive reception of health tech.

The multiplication of brilliant sensors and associated gadgets further extends the extent of wellbeing innovation. These sensors, implanted in regular items or coordinated into living conditions, catch an extensive variety of wellbeing related information without requiring unequivocal client input. Brilliant home gadgets, for example, can screen air quality, temperature, and even identify falls, adding to a more comprehensive comprehension of a singular's prosperity. The consistent joining of these sensor-based innovations into day to day existence obscures the lines between conventional medical services settings and the conditions individuals possess, making a ceaseless string of wellbeing checking all through different features of life.

Man-made consciousness and AI calculations assume a crucial part in opening the maximum capacity of health innovation. These cutting edge innovations, filled by tremendous datasets, can examine complex examples, foresee wellbeing results, and produce customized proposals. AI calculations filter through broad datasets to distinguish inconspicuous connections, empowering early location of medical problems and fitting mediations in view of individual wellbeing profiles. As computer based intelligence keeps on developing, its coordination into wellbeing tech vows to upset wellbeing checking by upgrading precision, prescient abilities, and the general adequacy of customized intercessions.

The shift towards proactive wellbeing the executives worked with by wellbeing innovation isn't restricted to individual clients; it reaches out to medical services frameworks and establishments. Distant Patient Checking (RPM) is acquiring conspicuousness, permitting medical care suppliers to screen patients' important bodily functions and wellbeing measurements outside customary clinical settings. This improves patient accommodation as well as empowers early location of weakening medical issue, diminishing the weight on medical care offices and possibly bringing down by and large medical care costs. The information created by wellbeing tech likewise adds to the advancement of proof based works on, empowering medical care suppliers to pursue more educated choices and designer mediations to individual necessities.

Moreover, the democratization of medical services is an eminent result of the wellbeing innovation upheaval. These advances separate geological boundaries, giving people in remote or underserved regions with apparatuses to screen and deal with their wellbeing. The openness of wellbeing related applications, wearables, and online stages rises above financial limits, engaging a different scope of people to proactively address their wellbeing concerns. This democratization lines up with the more extensive objective of accomplishing wellbeing value and guaranteeing that the advantages of innovative headways are open to all.

Regardless of the extraordinary capability of wellbeing innovation, it isn't invulnerable to difficulties and contemplations. Protection concerns encompassing the assortment and usage of individual wellbeing information are huge, provoking a basic assessment of information safety efforts and moral contemplations. Finding some kind of harmony between the advantages of customized wellbeing experiences and the security of individual protection is a squeezing worry that requires insightful administrative systems and straightforward correspondence from tech engineers.

Furthermore, the viability and exactness of health tech developments warrant progressing approval and refinement. While these advances hold gigantic commitment, guaranteeing their unwavering quality and exactness in assorted populaces and certifiable situations is urgent for laying out trust among clients and medical services experts the same.

Coordinated efforts between tech designers, medical care suppliers, and administrative bodies are fundamental for set powerful guidelines and guarantee that wellbeing tech meets the thorough necessities of the medical services scene.

As wellbeing innovation keeps on developing, its effect reaches out past individual wellbeing observing to impact general wellbeing drives and examination tries. The total of anonymized and collected information from enormous client bases sets out open doors for epidemiological investigations, sickness reconnaissance, and the ID of wellbeing patterns at a populace level. Saddling the force of wellbeing tech information on a more extensive scale can possibly illuminate general wellbeing approaches, shape preventive methodologies, and add to the progression of clinical information.

### 1.2 Historical perspective on the intersection of technology and health

The convergence of innovation and wellbeing is a dynamic and developing scene that has gone through critical changes throughout the span of history. From antiquated civic establishments to the current day, the connection among innovation and medical services has molded the manner in which social orders approach clinical practices, finding, therapy, and in general prosperity. Inspecting this verifiable viewpoint gives significant bits of knowledge into the direction of mechanical headways and their effect on the field of wellbeing.

In ancient history, different civic establishments created simple types of clinical innovation that mirrored comprehension they might interpret the human body and wellbeing. The old Egyptians, for example, utilized straightforward instruments like blades and tests for surgeries, while the Greeks utilized symptomatic techniques like palpation and perception. The restricted innovative instruments accessible during these times were a demonstration of the incipient condition of clinical information, with the accentuation put on all encompassing ways to deal with wellbeing that frequently consolidated profound and powerful components.

The Medieval times saw a steady change in the impression of wellbeing and the job of innovation in medication. With the appearance of imprinting in the fifteenth 100 years, clinical information turned out to be all the more broadly available through the scattering of books and original copies. This obvious the start of a more methodical documentation of clinical practices and the collection of information that laid the basis for future headways. Nonetheless, mechanical advancements in this period were still generally unassuming, and the comprehension of the human body remained affected by strict and philosophical convictions.

The Renaissance time saw a resurgence of interest in technical studies and a rejuvenation of clinical information. Mechanical progressions, like the improvement of additional modern careful instruments, started to assume a part in forming clinical practices. The development of the magnifying lens in the seventeenth hundred years by Anton van Leeuwenhoek opened new wildernesses in figuring out life systems and pathology at the phone level. This mechanical advancement made ready for huge advances in clinical exploration and established the groundwork for the areas of microbial science and pathology.

The nineteenth century saw a fast speed increase of mechanical development in medical services, energized by the Modern Unrest and a more deliberate way to deal with logical request. The creation of the stethoscope by René Laennec in 1816 reformed the determination of respiratory and cardiovascular circumstances, denoting the start of demonstrative apparatuses that were both harmless and mechanically progressed. The century likewise saw the improvement of sedation, making surgeries more okay for patients and taking into account more mind boggling mediations.

The last 50% of the nineteenth hundred years and the mid twentieth century were portrayed by the rise of X-beams and their application in clinical imaging. Wilhelm Roentgen's revelation of X-beams in 1895 changed the field of diagnostics, empowering doctors to imagine the inward designs of the human body without obtrusive strategies. This advancement significantly affected clinical work on, prompting more exact analyses and directing treatment choices.

The mid-twentieth century saw one more vital second with the improvement of anti-infection agents, for example, penicillin, which altered the treatment of bacterial diseases. The drug business assumed a focal part in this period, utilizing mechanical progressions in science and science to orchestrate and deliver new medications. The large scale manufacturing of anti-toxins denoted a defining moment in medical services, definitely lessening death rates from irresistible illnesses.

The last 50% of the twentieth hundred years and the mid 21st century saw the ascent of data innovation and its joining into medical care frameworks. The approach of electronic wellbeing records (EHRs) changed how clinical data was put away, got to, and shared. Computerized imaging advancements, for example, attractive reverberation imaging (X-ray) and processed tomography (CT) checks, gave clinicians phenomenal detail for finding and treatment arranging. The 1980s saw the improvement of the primary clinical imaging data frameworks, laying the basis for the digitalization of clinical records and pictures.

The late twentieth century likewise saw the rise of telemedicine, an idea that use media communications innovation to give medical care benefits from a distance.

While telemedicine has old roots as composed correspondence among doctors and patients, present day innovation has empowered continuous sound and video meetings, remote checking, and the trading of clinical data over tremendous distances. This has demonstrated particularly important in tending to medical care differences in rustic and underserved regions.

The 21st century has seen an extraordinary speed increase of mechanical development in medical care, with an emphasis on customized and preventive medication. The coming of genomics and the Human Genome Undertaking in the mid 2000s denoted a groundbreaking second, considering a more profound comprehension of hereditary elements impacting wellbeing and illness. This information has prepared for accuracy medication, where medicines are custom-made to a person's hereditary cosmetics, prompting more viable and designated mediations.

Wearable innovation has turned into a sign of the 21st-century crossing point of innovation and wellbeing. Gadgets, for example, smartwatches and wellness trackers furnished with sensors for checking pulse, rest designs, and actual work have enabled people to play a functioning job in their prosperity. The information gathered by these wearables not just furnishes clients with experiences into their wellbeing yet additionally adds to the accumulation of populace scale wellbeing information for examination and general wellbeing purposes.

Computerized reasoning (simulated intelligence) and AI have arisen as huge advantages in medical services, offering the possibility to break down immense measures of clinical information, distinguish examples, and make expectations. Man-made intelligence applications range from symptomatic devices and treatment suggestions to sedate revelation and customized wellbeing intercessions. The combination of man-made intelligence into medical services frameworks is ready to upgrade effectiveness, precision, and the general nature of care.

The Coronavirus pandemic, which started in 2019, highlighted the basic job of innovation in answering worldwide wellbeing emergencies. Telemedicine experienced exceptional development for the purpose of conveying medical care while limiting the gamble of viral transmission. Contact following applications and advanced wellbeing visas arose as apparatuses for following and dealing with the spread of the infection. The improvement of immunizations against the novel Covid was advanced through cutting edge biotechnological approaches and cooperative exploration endeavors, exhibiting the deftness of current innovation in tending to pressing medical services difficulties.

As innovation keeps on propelling, the convergence of innovation and wellbeing is ready for additional extraordinary turns of events. The mix of information from wearables, hereditary testing, and different sources into far reaching wellbeing profiles holds the commitment of conveying more customized and exact medical services. The continuous advancement of man-made intelligence and AI calculations is supposed to refine diagnostics, treatment methodologies, and prescient demonstrating.

Nonetheless, the fast speed of mechanical development likewise delivers moral, administrative, and social contemplations. Security concerns connected with the assortment and utilization of individual wellbeing information, the evenhanded appropriation of mechanical headways, and the potential for predisposition in computer based intelligence calculations are among the provokes that should be addressed as innovation keeps on molding the eventual fate of medical services.

### 1.3 Importance of health monitoring in the modern age

In the cutting edge age, the significance of wellbeing observing has become progressively obvious as social orders wrestle with the difficulties presented by a quickly changing medical services scene, developing ways of life, and the pervasiveness of ongoing sicknesses. Wellbeing observing, when a responsive practice held for clinical settings, has now changed into a proactive and constant undertaking worked with by progressions in innovation. This shift is supported by the acknowledgment that early recognition, customized mediations, and the strengthening of people in dealing with their wellbeing are fundamental parts of a vigorous medical services framework.

One of the essential drivers highlighting the significance of wellbeing observing is the rising weight of persistent sicknesses around the world. Conditions like diabetes, cardiovascular illnesses, and respiratory problems have arrived at pestilence extents, contributing essentially to grimness and mortality. Wellbeing checking assumes a significant part in the early recognition and the executives of these constant circumstances. Consistent following of key wellbeing pointers, for example, blood glucose levels, circulatory strain, and respiratory capability, permits people and medical care experts to distinguish deviations from ordinary reaches, empowering convenient intercessions to forestall difficulties and further develop results.

With regards to constant sickness the executives, wellbeing checking has developed past intermittent visits to medical care suppliers. The coming of wearable gadgets, for example, smartwatches and wellness trackers, has engaged people to screen their wellbeing progressively. These gadgets, outfitted with sensors that catch information on active work, pulse, rest examples, and the sky is the limit from there, furnish clients with a complete outline of their prosperity. The prompt admittance to such information cultivates a feeling of pride and mindfulness, empowering people to settle on informed conclusions about their way of life and wellbeing propensities.

The reconciliation of wellbeing checking into day to day existence isn't restricted to wearables; versatile applications likewise assume a significant part. Wellbeing and health applications act as incorporated stages for amassing and deciphering information from different sources, including wearables, permitting clients to follow patterns, put forth wellbeing objectives, and get customized suggestions. The consistent incorporation of wearables and applications into regular schedules changes wellbeing checking from an inconsistent movement into a nonstop, client driven insight.

Besides, wellbeing observing has turned into a vital part of preventive medical services methodologies. Perceiving that forestalling the beginning of illnesses is more viable and affordable than treating them, wellbeing frameworks and people the same are progressively focusing on preventive measures. Routine wellbeing screenings, inoculations, and way of life alterations directed by persistent observing add to early intercession and hazard decrease. The proactive idea of wellbeing observing lines up with a shift from the customary model of responsive medical care to a more all encompassing and expectant methodology.

In the period of data, where information driven bits of knowledge are forming different parts of society, wellbeing observing adds to the abundance of wellbeing related information. The total of anonymized and collected information from huge populaces sets out open doors for epidemiological examinations, general wellbeing research, and the distinguishing proof of wellbeing patterns. Tackling this information can illuminate general wellbeing approaches, help in the designation of assets, and add to the improvement of designated mediations to address explicit wellbeing challenges.

Mechanical headways, especially in the fields of man-made consciousness (man-made intelligence) and AI, have additionally raised the significance and abilities of wellbeing observing. These trend setting innovations can dissect immense datasets with exceptional speed and exactness, recognize designs, and create prescient models. In wellbeing checking, man-made intelligence calculations can help with deciphering complex information, foreseeing wellbeing results, and customizing mediations in view of individual wellbeing profiles. The reconciliation of simulated intelligence into wellbeing checking frameworks upgrades the proficiency and viability of medical care conveyance.

The Coronavirus pandemic, which has altogether affected social orders worldwide, plays highlighted the basic part of wellbeing checking in overseeing general wellbeing emergencies. Fast and broad testing, contact following, and checking of side effects have been fundamental parts of the reaction to the pandemic. Portable applications intended for Coronavirus contact following and side effect checking play had a urgent impact in recognizing and confining possible cases, moderating the spread of the infection. The pandemic has featured the requirement for hearty and versatile wellbeing checking frameworks that can answer arising dangers progressively.

In the work environment, wellbeing checking has acquired unmistakable quality as associations perceive the worth of representative prosperity for efficiency and generally hierarchical wellbeing. Corporate wellbeing programs frequently incorporate wellbeing observing parts, for example, wellness challenges, psychological well-being evaluations, and preventive screenings. Wearable gadgets might be incorporated into work environment health drives, permitting representatives to follow their actual work, screen feelings of anxiety, and get wellbeing tips. By advancing a culture of wellbeing and prosperity, businesses expect to upgrade worker fulfillment, lessen non-appearance, and work on by and large hierarchical execution.

Past individual and hierarchical advantages, wellbeing checking adds to the more extensive objectives of general wellbeing and medical services frameworks. Far off Quiet Observing (RPM) has arisen as a huge headway, permitting medical care suppliers to screen patients' important bodily functions and wellbeing measurements beyond conventional clinical settings. RPM is especially significant for people with constant circumstances, giving a nonstop stream of information that empowers ideal intercessions and lessens the requirement for incessant emergency clinic visits. This upgrades patient comfort as well as adds to more proficient medical services conveyance, advancing assets and further developing in general medical services results.

The significance of wellbeing checking is additionally emphasizd in the domain of maturing populaces. As socioeconomics shift towards more established age gatherings, the predominance old enough related conditions and the requirement for long haul care increment. Wellbeing checking advances, including savvy home gadgets, wearable sensors, and telehealth arrangements, offer the possibility to help maturing people in dealing with their wellbeing, keeping up with autonomy, and getting opportune clinical consideration. The capacity to screen essential signs, recognize falls, and survey by and large prosperity remotely becomes instrumental in giving viable and humane consideration to maturing populaces.

While the advantages of wellbeing checking are clear, it is vital to address difficulties and contemplations related with its execution. Security concerns connected with the assortment and utilization of individual wellbeing information are foremost. Finding some kind of harmony between bridling the capability of wellbeing observing and safeguarding individual security requires hearty administrative systems, straightforward correspondence, and moral contemplations. The turn of events and adherence to norms that guarantee the solid and moral utilization of wellbeing information are fundamental for cultivating trust among people and keeping up with the honesty of wellbeing observing frameworks.

Besides, the computerized partition represents a test to the evenhanded reception of wellbeing observing innovations. Financial variables, geological variations, and shifting degrees of mechanical education can make boundaries to get to. Guaranteeing that wellbeing checking arrangements are comprehensive and available to different populaces is fundamental for understanding the full advantages of these innovations. Cooperative endeavors between innovation engineers, medical services suppliers, policymakers, and local area partners are vital in addressing variations and elevating equivalent admittance to wellbeing observing assets.

# *Chapter 2*

## Wearable Devices and Health Tracking

Wearable gadgets and wellbeing following have become indispensable parts of the contemporary medical services scene, changing the manner in which people draw in with their prosperity. These innovations, going from smartwatches and wellness trackers to savvy clothing and implantable sensors, offer a range of elements intended to screen and improve different parts of wellbeing. The combination of wearables with cutting edge sensors, network, and information examination has introduced another time of customized, proactive medical care. In this investigation, we dive into the advancement, applications, difficulties, and future possibilities of wearable gadgets and wellbeing following.

**Development of Wearable Gadgets:**

The foundations of wearable innovation can be followed back to the early examinations with wristwatches and simple pedometers. Nonetheless, the groundbreaking jump happened in the 21st hundred years with the approach of scaled down sensors, low-power processors, and remote availability. These mechanical headways prepared for the advancement of wearables that could catch, process, and communicate wellbeing related information consistently.

The presentation of the principal wellness trackers in the last part of the 2000s denoted a huge achievement. These gadgets, frequently worn on the wrist, zeroed in fundamentally on observing active work, steps taken, and calories consumed. After some time, the capacities of wearables extended to incorporate pulse observing, rest following, and combination with cell phones for a more complete wellbeing checking experience.

Smartwatches arose as a noticeable class of wearables, consolidating wellbeing following highlights with the usefulness of customary watches and cell phone warnings. The combination of touchscreens, high level sensors, and adjustable applications changed smartwatches into flexible gadgets equipped for checking an expansive scope of wellbeing measurements.

Past wrist-worn gadgets, the scene of wearables reached out to incorporate brilliant dressing installed with sensors to screen indispensable signs, stance, and development. Also, implantable sensors, however more uncommon, have been investigated for applications, for example, ceaseless glucose observing for people with diabetes.

**Uses of Wearable Wellbeing Innovation:**

The uses of wearable wellbeing innovation are different, including different features of physical and mental prosperity. The most common functionalities include:

**Movement Following:** Wearables act as modern pedometers, following advances, distance voyaged, and in general actual work. These elements are fundamental for advancing a functioning way of life and forestalling inactive way of behaving.

**Pulse Checking:** Consistent pulse observing gives bits of knowledge into cardiovascular wellbeing, empowering clients to follow their resting pulse, identify oddities, and measure their wellness levels.

**Rest Following:** Wearables outfitted with rest following capacities screen rest examples, length, and quality. This data helps clients in streamlining their rest cleanliness and distinguishing potential rest issues.

**Stress The executives:** A few wearables integrate sensors to gauge feelings of anxiety in view of physiological pointers, for example, pulse changeability. Clients get input and proposals for stress decrease strategies.

**Caloric Admission and Use:** High level wearables might coordinate with nourishment following applications, permitting clients to screen their caloric admission and consumption. This element supports weight the executives and advances a fair eating routine.

**Pulse Observing:** Certain wearables, especially those with cutting edge sensors, offer circulatory strain checking abilities, giving clients bits of knowledge into their vascular wellbeing.

**Older Consideration and Fall Discovery:** Wearables furnished with accelerometers and spinners can be instrumental in old consideration, offering fall identification includes that ready parental figures or crisis administrations in case of a fall.

**Ongoing Illness The board:** Wearables assume a critical part in overseeing constant circumstances like diabetes. Nonstop glucose observing, for instance, permits people to screen their glucose levels progressively.

**Conceptive Wellbeing Following:** A few wearables take care of ladies' wellbeing by offering highlights for feminine cycle following, ovulation expectation, and richness checking.

**Biofeedback and Care:** Wearables with biofeedback abilities work with care and stress decrease through directed breathing activities and unwinding strategies.

These applications all in all add to a comprehensive comprehension of a singular's wellbeing, cultivating a proactive way to deal with prosperity.

**Difficulties and Contemplations:**

Regardless of the bunch advantages of wearable gadgets and wellbeing following, a few difficulties and contemplations merit consideration:

**Protection and Security Concerns:** The assortment and capacity of individual wellbeing information raise protection concerns. Guaranteeing powerful safety efforts and straightforward information taking care of practices is fundamental for fabricate client trust.

**Information Exactness and Dependability:** The precision of sensor readings and information understanding is basic for the believability of wellbeing experiences given by wearables. Alignment, approval, and adherence to quality norms are fundamental.

**Interoperability and Normalization:** The similarity of wearables with different gadgets and stages, as well as the normalization of information designs, remain difficulties. Consistent reconciliation with electronic wellbeing records and medical services frameworks is urgent for far reaching wellbeing the board.

**Client Adherence and Commitment:** Supporting client commitment over the long haul is a typical test. Wearables need to offer significant bits of knowledge, noteworthy suggestions, and a natural client experience to keep people persuaded.

**Battery Duration and Gadget Sturdiness:** The restricted battery duration of numerous wearables can be a deterrent. Improvements in battery innovation and gadget toughness are fundamental for delayed and solid use.

**Moral Contemplations:** The moral ramifications of wearables, for example, the potential for information abuse or separation in view of wellbeing measurements, require cautious thought. It is basic to Lay out moral rules and guidelines.

**Reasonableness and Availability:** The expense of top of the line wearables might restrict their openness to specific socioeconomics. Guaranteeing reasonableness and tending to abberations in access are essential for far reaching reception.

**Medical services Proficient Combination:** Really coordinating wearable produced information into medical services work processes and working with joint effort among clients and medical services experts is fundamental for amplifying the effect of wellbeing following.

**Approval and Clinical Viability:** Showing the clinical adequacy of wearables in forestalling and overseeing ailments is a continuous test. Thorough examination and approval studies are important to lay out the dependability and adequacy of wellbeing following elements.

**Client Schooling and Proficiency:** Advancing wellbeing proficiency and teaching clients on the translation of wellbeing information is fundamental. Errors or misinterpretations of information could prompt superfluous tension or deficient reaction to wellbeing markers.

Tending to these difficulties requires a cooperative exertion including innovation designers, medical services experts, policymakers, and clients to make an environment that focuses on the moral, precise, and client driven utilization of wearable wellbeing innovation.

**Future Possibilities:**

The eventual fate of wearable gadgets and wellbeing following holds massive potential, driven by continuous mechanical progressions and an advancing medical care scene:

**High level Sensor Advances:** Proceeded with headways in sensor innovations, including scaling down, further developed exactness, and the combination of new sensor modalities, will upgrade the capacities of wearables for more thorough wellbeing checking.

**Wearables as Clinical Gadgets:** Administrative organizations are progressively perceiving the clinical capability of specific wearables. A few gadgets are getting endorsement as clinical gadgets, showing a shift toward all the more clinically approved and controlled wellbeing following arrangements.

**Joining with Telehealth and Remote Observing:** Wearables will assume a focal part in the combination of telehealth and remote checking arrangements. These advancements work with persistent medical services conveyance, particularly for people with constant circumstances or those living in far off regions.

**Man-made reasoning and Prescient Examination:** The joining of man-made consciousness and AI calculations will empower wearables to give more customized and prescient wellbeing experiences. These calculations can dissect huge datasets to distinguish designs, anticipate wellbeing patterns, and propose custom-made proposals.

**Extended Applications in Emotional well-being:** Wearables will progressively zero in on emotional wellness following, offering highlights for pressure the board, state of mind checking, and rest quality appraisal. This comprehensive methodology perceives the interconnectedness of physical and mental prosperity.

**Brilliant Textures and Implantable Gadgets:** The improvement of savvy textures with installed sensors and implantable gadgets will grow the choices for wellbeing observing. These developments might give inconspicuous and ceaseless observing to different wellbeing boundaries.

**Blockchain for Information Security:** Blockchain innovation might be utilized to upgrade the security and honesty of wellbeing information created by wearables. Decentralized and secure information stockpiling could address protection concerns and work with interoperability.

**Customization and Personalization:** Wearables will progressively offer customization choices to take special care of individual inclinations and wellbeing objectives. Customized criticism and proposals in view of a singular's extraordinary wellbeing profile will improve client commitment.

**Hybrid with Expanded Reality (AR) and Augmented Reality (VR):** The assembly of wearables with AR and VR advancements could bring about imaginative answers for medical services training, helpful intercessions, and vivid wellbeing encounters.

**Epidemiological Exploration and General Wellbeing Effect:** The enormous scope information created by wearables hold extraordinary potential for epidemiological examination. Accumulated and anonymized information could add to the distinguishing proof of wellbeing patterns, infection areas of interest, and the advancement of designated general wellbeing intercessions.

As wearables keep on advancing, their part in molding the eventual fate of medical services is ready to grow. The continuous joint effort between innovation designers, medical care experts, scientists, and administrative bodies is critical for understanding the maximum capacity of wearables in advancing individual prosperity, forestalling illnesses, and adding to progressions in general wellbeing.

## 2.1 Exploration of popular wearable devices (smartwatches, fitness trackers, etc.)

The investigation of famous wearable gadgets, including smartwatches, wellness trackers, and other wellbeing driven innovations, divulges a different scene that has reshaped how people draw in with their wellbeing and prosperity. These gadgets, furnished with cutting edge sensors, network highlights, and easy to use interfaces, have become fundamental devices for wellbeing observing, movement following, and generally way of life the board. In this investigation, we dig into the elements, functionalities, and effect of probably the most famous wearable gadgets, featuring their commitments to the developing worldview of individual wellbeing the board.

**Smartwatches:**

**Outline:**

Smartwatches have arisen as multifunctional gadgets that join conventional timekeeping with a set-up of shrewd elements. They act as an expansion of cell phones, offering clients a helpful method for getting to notices, messages, and applications straightforwardly from their wrists. Notwithstanding their correspondence and efficiency capabilities, smartwatches have become strong wellbeing and wellness colleagues, coordinating sensors that screen different wellbeing measurements.

**Wellbeing and Wellness Highlights:**

Present day smartwatches are furnished with a variety of sensors to follow actual work, pulse, rest examples, and then some. The consideration of GPS usefulness takes into account precise following of open air exercises like running or cycling. Numerous smartwatches additionally offer water obstruction, making them appropriate for following swimming meetings.

**Wellbeing Checking:**

Smartwatches succeed in consistent wellbeing observing. They give continuous information on pulse, empowering clients to check their cardiovascular wellbeing and recognize peculiarities. A few models offer electrocardiogram (ECG or EKG) usefulness, permitting clients to record and examine their heart's electrical movement. This element can support identifying sporadic heart rhythms like atrial fibrillation.

**Rest Following:**

Rest following is one more unmistakable component in smartwatches. By observing development examples and pulse during rest, these gadgets give bits of knowledge into rest span, rest stages, and generally speaking rest quality. Clients can use this data to make way of life changes and further develop their rest cleanliness.

**Wellness and Exercise:**

Smartwatches act as thorough wellness partners, offering devoted modes for different activities. They track measurements, for example, steps taken, distance covered, calories consumed, and dynamic minutes. A few models go further by giving directed exercises, training, and execution examination. These highlights add to a more comprehensive way to deal with wellness the executives.

**Coordination with Wellbeing Applications:**

Smartwatches frequently coordinate with wellbeing and wellness applications, making a consistent biological system for clients. This coordination takes into consideration the accumulation of wellbeing information, customized bits of knowledge, and objective following. Clients can interface their smartwatches to stages that offer more extensive wellbeing and health administrations, cultivating a far reaching way to deal with wellbeing the board.

**Distant Wellbeing Checking:**

As of late, smartwatches play had an impact in far off wellbeing checking. With highlights like fall location and crisis SOS works, these gadgets can caution crisis contacts or administrations in case of a potential wellbeing emergency. This usefulness upgrades the security and prosperity of clients, especially those in danger of falls or other wellbeing crises.

**Wellness Trackers:**

**Outline:**

Wellness trackers, otherwise called movement trackers, are specific wearables planned principally for checking active work and advancing a solid way of life. While they might come up short on broad highlights of smartwatches, wellness trackers succeed in conveying precise and centered information connected with exercise and day to day development.

**Action Following:**

The center capability of wellness trackers is to screen everyday action. They count steps taken, gauge distance voyaged, and work out calories consumed in light of client development. This data gives clients a pattern comprehension of their everyday actual work and urges them to meet movement objectives.

**Pulse Checking:**

Numerous wellness trackers incorporate pulse checking capacities, empowering clients to follow their pulse during different exercises and over the course of the day. Persistent pulse observing adds to a more exact evaluation of by and large cardiovascular wellbeing and exercise force.

**Rest Following:**

Like smartwatches, wellness trackers frequently incorporate rest following highlights. By observing rest length, dissecting rest designs, and giving bits of knowledge into rest quality, these gadgets assist clients with laying out better rest schedules and distinguish factors that might influence their rest.

**Practice Modes:**

Wellness trackers offer predefined practice modes custom-made to explicit exercises like running, cycling, or weightlifting. Initiating these modes permits the gadget to give more precise information connected with the picked work out, including measurements like speed, term, and force.

**Objective Setting and Gamification:**

To inspire clients, wellness trackers frequently consolidate objective setting highlights and gamification components. Clients can define day to day or week by week movement objectives, and the tracker gives input and prizes after accomplishing these objectives. This gamified approach upgrades client commitment and energizes a more dynamic way of life.

**Moderateness and Long Battery Duration:**

One of the eminent benefits of wellness trackers is their moderateness contrasted with some smartwatches. Furthermore, wellness trackers normally gloat longer battery duration, in some cases enduring a few days on a solitary charge. This life span improves their convenience for consistent action following without regular re-energizing.

**Shrewd Dress:**

**Outline:**

Shrewd dress addresses a combination of innovation and materials, inserting sensors and conductive materials straightforwardly into pieces of clothing. This classification incorporates things like shrewd shirts, sports bras, and pressure pieces of clothing, which offer attentive wellbeing checking capacities without the requirement for extra frill.

**Biometric Checking:**

Shrewd dress consolidates sensors that screen different biometric markers, including pulse, respiratory rate, and internal heat level. The sensors are flawlessly woven into the texture, considering ceaseless and unpretentious checking during different exercises.

**Pose Revision and Development Investigation:**

Some shrewd dress things are intended to investigate stance and body development. These articles of clothing utilize implanted sensors to recognize changes in body situating and give criticism to clients, advancing better stance and structure during activities or everyday exercises.

**Launderable and Agreeable Plan:**

Shrewd attire is intended to be launderable and happy with, guaranteeing that the coordination of innovation doesn't think twice about piece of clothing's usefulness or wearability. The launderable idea of these articles of clothing recognizes them from numerous customary wearable gadgets that might require evacuation of electronic parts prior to cleaning.

**Applications in Medical services:**

Past wellness and wellbeing, savvy clothing has applications in medical care. For instance, articles of clothing furnished with sensors can be utilized for constant checking of patients with persistent circumstances, permitting medical services suppliers to assemble continuous information from a distance.

**Joining with Portable Applications:**

Savvy clothing things frequently incorporate with committed versatile applications to give clients an extensive perspective on their wellbeing measurements. These applications might offer elements, for example, authentic information examination, objective following, and customized proposals in view of the gathered information.

**Hearables (Shrewd Headphones):**

**Outline:**

Hearables, a class that incorporates savvy headphones, join sound functionalities with wellbeing checking highlights. These gadgets influence the nearness to the client's ears to catch physiological information and convey customized wellbeing experiences.

**Pulse Observing and Biometric Following:**

Shrewd headphones frequently incorporate optical sensors that action pulse through the veins in the ear. This gives a nonstop and unpretentious technique for checking pulse during different exercises, including exercises and everyday schedules.

**Action Following and Movement Sensors:**

Some hearables integrate movement sensors to follow active work, including steps taken and calories consumed. This component, joined with pulse checking, offers a more thorough outline of the client's day to day development and exercise designs.

**Ongoing Instructing and Input:**

Hearables with wellbeing following abilities might offer continuous instructing and criticism. For instance, during an exercise, the savvy miniature headphones can give direction on keeping an ideal pulse zone, right structure, or changing the power of the activity.

**Coordination with Remote helpers:**

Many shrewd headphones coordinate with menial helpers, empowering clients to get to wellbeing data, put forth wellbeing objectives, or get health tips through voice orders. This incorporation upgrades the general client experience and works with sans hands association.

**Hearing Wellbeing Observing:**

Notwithstanding wellness related highlights, some hearables center around observing hearing wellbeing. They can survey openness to boisterous sounds, give proposals to safeguard hearing, and track changes in hearing limits over the long haul.

**Difficulties and Contemplations:**

In spite of the exceptional progressions in wearable gadgets, a few difficulties and contemplations persevere in the domain of wellbeing observing wearables:

**Exactness and Dependability:** Guaranteeing the precision and unwavering quality of wellbeing measurements is principal. Changeability in sensor precision and information translation can affect the validity of wellbeing bits of knowledge given by wearables.

**Protection and Security:** The assortment, stockpiling, and transmission of wellbeing information raise critical protection and security concerns. Safeguarding client information from unapproved access and guaranteeing secure information taking care of practices are basic contemplations.

**Client Adherence:** Supporting client commitment over the drawn out stays a test.

Wearables need to give significant bits of knowledge, noteworthy proposals, and an instinctive client experience to keep people spurred.

**Interoperability:** The interoperability of wearables with different gadgets and stages, as well as the normalization of information designs, requires consideration. Consistent coordination with electronic wellbeing records and medical care frameworks is urgent for exhaustive wellbeing the board.

**Moral Contemplations:** The moral ramifications of wearables, including information possession, assent, and likely abuse of wellbeing information, request cautious thought. It is fundamental to Lay out moral rules and guidelines.

**Moderateness and Openness:** The expense of wearables, particularly top of the line gadgets, may restrict their availability to specific socioeconomics. Guaranteeing moderateness and tending to variations in access are vital for boundless reception.

**Battery Duration and Strength:** The restricted battery duration of numerous wearables and worries about gadget toughness remain contemplations. Upgrades in battery innovation and strong plan are fundamental for delayed and dependable use.

**Administrative Consistence:** Guaranteeing administrative consistence, especially for wearables with wellbeing observing highlights, is basic. Getting essential endorsements and sticking to norms upgrade the believability and wellbeing of these gadgets.

**Client Instruction:** Advancing client training on the understanding of wellbeing information and the legitimate utilization of wearables is fundamental. False impressions or misinterpretations of information could prompt superfluous nervousness or insufficient reactions to wellbeing markers.

**2.2 In-depth analysis of health tracking features, including heart rate monitoring, sleep tracking,**
**and activity tracking**

An inside and out investigation of wellbeing following elements, including pulse observing, rest following, and action following, uncovers the extraordinary effect of wearable gadgets and wellbeing advances on private prosperity. These elements, frequently coordinated into smartwatches, wellness trackers, and other wellbeing driven wearables, enable clients with constant experiences into their physiological measurements and everyday exercises. This extensive investigation investigates the importance, headways, difficulties, and future possibilities of these key wellbeing following highlights.

**Pulse Observing:**
**Importance and Headways:**
Pulse observing stands as a foundation of wellbeing following, giving a persistent evaluation of cardiovascular wellbeing. The meaning of observing pulse lies in its job as an essential sign of generally prosperity and wellness. Headways in wearable innovation have prompted the coordination of optical sensors that catch pulse information through photoplethysmography (PPG), empowering painless and constant observing.

Persistent pulse checking offers a few benefits, permitting clients to follow their resting pulse, notice patterns during active work, and recognize inconsistencies in pulse designs. A few wearable gadgets make this a stride further by giving bits of knowledge into pulse changeability (HRV), which mirrors the variety in time between progressive pulses. HRV is related with autonomic sensory system movement and can offer experiences into feelings of anxiety and by and large cardiovascular wellbeing.

**Wellness and Exercise Enhancement:**

For wellness lovers and competitors, pulse observing assumes an essential part in improving preparation regimens. Wearables furnished with pulse sensors give measurements, for example, target pulse zones, permitting clients to tailor their exercises to accomplish explicit wellness objectives. By remaining inside the ideal pulse range during exercise, people can amplify the productivity of their exercises and improve cardiovascular wellness.

**Wellbeing Experiences and Inconsistency Recognition:**

Nonstop pulse observing adds to the early recognition of potential medical problems. Wearables can make clients aware of strange pulse designs, for example, supported high or low pulses, which might show conditions like atrial fibrillation or bradycardia. This proactive observing ability engages clients to look for clinical consideration immediately, possibly forestalling more serious unexpected problems.

**Stress The executives:**

A few wearables influence pulse information to give experiences into feelings of anxiety. Pulse changeability, specifically, is associated with the body's reaction to stretch. By dissecting designs in HRV, wearables can offer criticism on feelings of anxiety and, at times, give directed breathing activities or care exercises to advance unwinding.

**Rest Following:**

**Importance and Headways:**

Rest following has arisen as an important wellbeing following component, perceiving the fundamental job of value rest in generally speaking prosperity. Wearables with rest following capacities utilize a blend of accelerometer information and pulse observing to evaluate rest examples, length, and quality. High level rest following elements plan to give clients significant bits of knowledge to further develop their rest cleanliness.

**Rest Length and Examples:**

One of the key measurements presented by rest following is all out rest term. Wearables examine development designs during the night to decide times of tranquil rest and attentiveness. By understanding rest length, clients can evaluate whether they are meeting prescribed rest rules and make changes in accordance with focus on sufficient rest.

**Rest Stages:**

Wearables furnished with cutting edge rest following can separate between rest stages, including light rest, profound rest, and REM (quick eye development) rest. Each stage serves particular physiological capabilities, and understanding the creation of rest stages gives clients experiences into the general nature of their rest.

**Rest Quality Measurements:**

Notwithstanding span and stages, wearables frequently give measurements characteristic of rest quality. These measurements might incorporate rest productivity, which estimates the level of time invested snoozing contrasted with energy spent in bed, and rest beginning idleness, which addresses the time it takes to nod off. By surveying these measurements, clients can distinguish factors influencing the general nature of their rest.

**Rest Climate Examination:**

A few wearables consolidate natural sensors to examine factors in the rest climate, like room temperature, encompassing light, and commotion levels. This extra information adds to a more far reaching comprehension of the variables impacting rest quality and assists clients with making acclimations to establish a favorable rest climate.

**Savvy Alert Elements:**

To upgrade the waking experience, many rest following wearables incorporate shrewd caution highlights. These highlights plan to wake clients during a light rest stage, limiting the sluggishness related with waking from profound rest. By synchronizing the caution with the client's rest cycle, wearables mean to advance a more regular and reviving waking experience.

**Movement Following:**

**Importance and Headways:**

Movement following is a basic wellbeing observing element that tends to the stationary idea of present day ways of life. The importance lies in empowering people to embrace a more dynamic and better lifestyle. Headways in action following have developed past straightforward step counting, consolidating a scope of measurements to give a comprehensive perspective on day to day active work.

**Step Counting and Distance Estimation:**

The essential part of action following is step counting, which measures the quantity of stages a singular requires over the course of the day. Wearables with accelerometers precisely measure steps, permitting clients to put forth and track day to day step objectives. Distance estimation, frequently got from step count and step length, gives an extra measurement to checking generally speaking development.

**Caloric Use:**

Movement trackers gauge caloric consumption in light of elements, for example, step count, action power, and client profile data. This measurement assists people with understanding the energy used during different exercises, adding to a more educated way to deal with adjusting energy admission and use.

**Dynamic Minutes and Force Levels:**

To advance a more nuanced comprehension of active work, wearables present measurements, for example, dynamic minutes and power levels. Dynamic minutes evaluate times of moderate to lively actual work, offering experiences into the span of exercises that add to cardiovascular wellness. Power levels sort movement into zones, like light, moderate, and overwhelming, giving a more itemized investigation of activity force.

**Reconciliation with Exercise Modes:**
Wearables take care of different activity inclinations by offering devoted modes for explicit exercises like running, cycling, swimming, and weightlifting. Initiating these modes upgrades the precision of measurements connected with the picked work out, giving clients nitty gritty experiences into their exhibition and progress.

**Objective Setting and Gamification:**
Movement following wearables frequently integrate objective setting elements to propel clients. Defining day to day or week after week objectives for steps, distance, or dynamic minutes gives people a substantial objective to pursue. Gamification components, for example, accomplishment identifications or virtual prizes, upgrade client commitment and encourage a feeling of achievement.

**Social and Local area Reconciliation:**
To upgrade inspiration and responsibility, numerous action following wearables include social and local area mix. Clients can interface with companions, join difficulties, and offer their accomplishments. The social viewpoint establishes a strong climate, cultivating solid rivalry and empowering people to remain dynamic.

**Difficulties and Contemplations:**
While wellbeing following elements have achieved huge progressions in private prosperity, a few difficulties and contemplations warrant consideration:

**Exactness and Unwavering quality:** Guaranteeing the precision and dependability of wellbeing following measurements is significant for building client trust. Fluctuation in sensor exactness and information translation can affect the validity of wellbeing bits of knowledge given by wearables.

**Individual Fluctuation:** Wellbeing following measurements are dependent upon individual changeability. Factors, for example, age, wellness level, and ailments can impact the translation of information. Wearables need to represent these factors to give significant and customized bits of knowledge.

**Protection and Security:** The assortment, stockpiling, and transmission of wellbeing information raise critical security and security concerns. Safeguarding client information from unapproved access and guaranteeing secure information dealing with rehearses are basic contemplations.

**Client Adherence:** Supporting client commitment over the drawn out stays a test. Wearables need to give significant bits of knowledge, noteworthy proposals, and an instinctive client experience to keep people propelled.

**Interoperability:** The interoperability of wearables with different gadgets and stages, as well as the normalization of information designs, requires consideration. Consistent joining with electronic wellbeing records and medical care frameworks is vital for exhaustive wellbeing the board.

**Moral Contemplations:** The moral ramifications of wearables, including information possession, assent, and likely abuse of wellbeing information, request cautious thought. It is fundamental to Lay out moral rules and guidelines.

**Reasonableness and Openness:** The expense of wearables, particularly top of the line gadgets, may restrict their availability to specific socioeconomics. Guaranteeing moderateness and tending to differences in access are significant for far reaching reception.

**Client Schooling:** Advancing client instruction on the translation of wellbeing information and the legitimate utilization of wearables is fundamental. Mistaken assumptions or misinterpretations of information could prompt superfluous uneasiness or insufficient reactions to wellbeing pointers.

**Future Possibilities:**

The fate of wellbeing following elements holds energizing prospects, driven by continuous mechanical progressions and a developing accentuation on customized, preventive medical care:

**High level Sensor Advancements:** Proceeded with progressions in sensor advances, including the coordination of new sensor modalities, will improve the exactness and scope of wellbeing following elements. Scaling down and further developed sensor responsiveness will add to more refined observing abilities.

**Reconciliation with Man-made reasoning (computer based intelligence):** The combination of man-made reasoning and AI calculations will empower wearables to give more customized and prescient wellbeing bits of knowledge. These calculations can break down immense datasets to recognize designs, foresee wellbeing patterns, and present custom-made suggestions.

**Wearable ECG and Circulatory strain Checking:** Wearables with ECG and pulse observing abilities will turn out to be more predominant. These elements, when selective to clinical grade gadgets, will offer clients more far reaching cardiovascular wellbeing observing.

**Biometric Validation:** Wellbeing following wearables might advance to incorporate biometric verification highlights, utilizing extraordinary physiological measurements, for example, pulse changeability for secure and consistent client recognizable proof.

**Extended Emotional wellness Following:** The mix of psychological well-being following elements, including feelings of anxiety, state of mind examples, and rest quality, will turn out to be more refined. Wearables will assume an expanded part in advancing all encompassing prosperity, tending to the interconnectedness of physical and psychological well-being.

**Natural and Context oriented Experiences:** Wearables might integrate ecological sensors to give context oriented bits of knowledge into elements like air quality, temperature, and UV openness. This extra information can add to a more far reaching comprehension of wellbeing powerhouses.

**Blockchain for Information Security:** Blockchain innovation might be utilized to upgrade the security and honesty of wellbeing information created by wearables. Decentralized and secure information stockpiling could address protection concerns and work with interoperability.

**Customization and Personalization:** Wearables will progressively offer customization choices to take special care of individual inclinations and wellbeing objectives.

Customized criticism and proposals in view of a singular's one of a kind wellbeing profile will upgrade client commitment.

**Coordination with Telehealth:** The combination of wearables with telehealth stages will work with remote checking and virtual medical care meetings. Wearables will become indispensable instruments for telehealth suppliers, offering constant wellbeing information for more educated navigation.

**Epidemiological Exploration:** Amassed and anonymized information from wearables hold incredible potential for epidemiological examination. Enormous scope information examination could add to the ID of wellbeing patterns, sickness areas of interest, and the improvement of designated general wellbeing intercessions.

As wellbeing following highlights keep on advancing, the cooperative endeavors of innovation designers, medical care experts, specialists, and administrative bodies will be vital for tackling the maximum capacity of wearables. By tending to difficulties, guaranteeing precision, and focusing on client driven plan, wellbeing following wearables can assume a focal part in forming the fate of medical care — a future portrayed by customized, proactive, and interconnected ways to deal with prosperity.

### 2.3 Highlighting the impact of wearables on personal health and fitness

Wearables have arisen as useful assets that altogether influence individual wellbeing and wellness, altering the manner in which people approach health. These gadgets, going from smartwatches and wellness trackers to savvy clothing and hearables, are furnished with cutting edge sensors, network elements, and wellbeing following capacities. The effect of wearables on private wellbeing and wellness is diverse, impacting regions like active work, cardiovascular wellbeing, rest quality, and by and large way of life the executives.

**Empowering Actual work:**

One of the most remarkable effects of wearables is their capacity to spur and energize actual work. Through highlights like step counting, distance following, and dynamic minutes checking, wearables give people unmistakable measurements that evaluate their day to day development. This information fills in as a persuasive device, empowering clients to put forth and accomplish movement objectives. The gamification components integrated into numerous wearables, like virtual identifications and difficulties, further improve client commitment, cultivating a feeling of achievement and solid contest.

By advancing a more dynamic way of life, wearables add to the counteraction of stationary way of behaving — a critical gamble factor for different medical issue, including cardiovascular infection, corpulence, and diabetes. The ongoing input and objective setting highlights enable people to go with cognizant decisions to build their day to day actual work, eventually further developing their general wellness levels.

**Thorough Wellbeing Observing:**

Wearables go past fundamental movement following, offering thorough wellbeing checking abilities. One of the key effects is in the domain of cardiovascular wellbeing.

With nonstop pulse checking and, now and again, electrocardiogram (ECG or EKG) usefulness, wearables give clients experiences into their heart wellbeing.

Checking resting pulse, identifying oddities, and surveying pulse fluctuation add to a more comprehensive comprehension of cardiovascular prosperity.

The effect of wearables stretches out to rest quality, a basic part of generally wellbeing. High level rest following elements examine rest span, stages, and quality. By giving people significant experiences into their rest designs, wearables enable clients to make way of life changes that decidedly influence their rest. Further developed rest quality improves actual recuperation as well as has significant ramifications for psychological well-being and mental capability.

**Advancing Customized Wellness:**

Wearables assume a critical part in advancing customized wellness regimens. The coordination of activity modes for different exercises, like running, cycling, and strength preparing, permits clients to fit their exercises to their inclinations and wellness objectives. Wearables give constant measurements during exercise, including pulse, power levels, and length, empowering clients to streamline their instructional courses for most extreme effectiveness.

The effect of wearables on customized wellness is additionally exemplified by their capacity to adjust to individual wellness levels and progress. As clients reliably draw in with their wearables, these gadgets gain from their action examples and present progressively exact suggestions and bits of knowledge. This versatile methodology guarantees that wellness direction stays applicable and testing, supporting consistent improvement and forestalling leveling.

**Stress The board and Prosperity:**

The combination of stress checking highlights in wearables tends to the all encompassing nature of wellbeing and prosperity. By utilizing pulse fluctuation and other physiological pointers, wearables offer experiences into feelings of anxiety and, in certain examples, give directed unwinding activities or care exercises. This effect on pressure the board lines up with the developing acknowledgment of the interconnectedness of physical and psychological well-being.

Persistent pressure has significant ramifications for wellbeing, adding to conditions like hypertension, sleep deprivation, and compromised invulnerable capability. Wearables, by working with pressure mindfulness and offering devices for stress decrease, engage people to proactively deal with their psychological prosperity. The effect of wearables in such manner reaches out past simple wellness following, situating them as all encompassing wellbeing friends that address the unpredictable connection among physical and psychological well-being.

**Upgraded Responsibility and Inspiration:**

Wearables present a layer of responsibility and inspiration that fundamentally influences people's adherence to wellbeing and wellness objectives. The continuous idea of criticism, combined with objective setting highlights and updates, keeps clients effectively took part in their wellbeing process. The effect of wearables on responsibility is increased by the social and local area combination includes that permit clients to associate with companions, join difficulties, and offer their accomplishments.

The social part of wearables changes wellbeing and wellness into a collective encounter, encouraging a strong climate. Whether through virtual contests or cooperative difficulties, people track down inspiration in the common quest for prosperity. This shared effect reaches out to the domain of responsibility, as the information that others know about one's wellbeing and wellness objectives makes a feeling of obligation and responsibility.

**Consistent Observing and Early Discovery:**

The consistent observing capacities of wearables add to early location and proactive administration of medical problems. The effect on early identification is especially obvious in cardiovascular wellbeing. Wearables furnished with cutting edge sensors can recognize unpredictable pulse designs, possibly flagging circumstances like atrial fibrillation. This early location engages clients to look for clinical consideration quickly, working with opportune intercessions and decreasing the gamble of intricacies.

Furthermore, wearables might assume a part in far off wellbeing checking, particularly for people with ongoing circumstances. The constant transmission of wellbeing information to medical care suppliers empowers proactive administration and convenient acclimations to therapy plans. This effect on constant checking lines up with the more extensive shift towards preventive medical care, where early discovery and intercession are focused on to further develop wellbeing results.

**Difficulties and Contemplations:**

While the effect of wearables on private wellbeing and wellness is significant, a few difficulties and contemplations merit consideration:

**Exactness and Unwavering quality:** Guaranteeing the precision and dependability of wellbeing measurements is principal for client trust. Changeability in sensor exactness and information translation can affect the validity of wellbeing experiences given by wearables.

**Protection and Security:** The assortment, stockpiling, and transmission of wellbeing information raise critical security and security concerns. Safeguarding client information from unapproved access and guaranteeing secure information dealing with rehearses are basic contemplations.

**Client Adherence:** Supporting client commitment over the drawn out stays a test. Wearables need to give significant bits of knowledge, noteworthy suggestions, and an instinctive client experience to keep people persuaded.

**Interoperability:** The interoperability of wearables with different gadgets and stages, as well as the normalization of information designs, requires consideration. Consistent incorporation with electronic wellbeing records and medical care frameworks is essential for extensive wellbeing the executives.

**Moral Contemplations:** The moral ramifications of wearables, including information possession, assent, and expected abuse of wellbeing information, request cautious thought. It is fundamental to Lay out moral rules and guidelines.

**Moderateness and Availability:** The expense of wearables, particularly very good quality gadgets, may restrict their openness to specific socioeconomics. Guaranteeing reasonableness and tending to abberations in access are essential for boundless reception.

# Chapter 3

**Remote Patient Monitoring**

Distant Patient Checking (RPM) addresses a groundbreaking way to deal with medical care conveyance, utilizing innovation to screen patients outside conventional clinical settings. This change in perspective holds the possibility to upgrade patient results, lessen medical services costs, and work on the general nature of care. As the medical services scene keeps on developing, the reception of RPM is picking up speed, driven by progressions in advanced wellbeing innovations and the developing accentuation on tolerant driven care. This thorough investigation digs into the complexities of Far off Understanding Checking, analyzing its applications, advantages, difficulties, and future possibilities.

1. **Prologue to Distant Patient Observing:**
   Distant Patient Observing is a medical services methodology that utilizes innovation to gather patient information beyond ordinary medical services settings and send it to medical care suppliers for evaluation and mediation. The objective is to screen patients progressively, empowering proactive administration of ongoing circumstances, early identification of expected issues, and convenient mediations, all while engaging patients to take part in their consideration effectively.

   The underpinning of RPM lies in the use of different advanced wellbeing apparatuses and gadgets, including wearable sensors, savvy gadgets, versatile applications, and telehealth stages. These innovations work with the consistent checking of indispensable signs, side effects, and other significant wellbeing measurements, making a dynamic and interconnected medical services environment.

2. **Key Parts of Distant Patient Checking:**
   **Wearable Gadgets and Sensors:**
   Wearable gadgets furnished with sensors structure an essential part of RPM. These gadgets, which can incorporate smartwatches, wellness trackers, and

clinical grade wearables, catch physiological information, for example, pulse, circulatory strain, oxygen immersion, and action levels. Wearables offer a non-meddling and helpful method for persistent observing, permitting patients to approach their day to day routines while producing significant wellbeing information.

**Remote Checking Stages:**

The foundation supporting RPM includes vigorous remote checking stages. These stages act as the focal center for gathering, putting away, and breaking down tolerant produced information. Mix with electronic wellbeing records (EHRs) and other medical services frameworks guarantees consistent correspondence between remote checking stages and the more extensive medical services foundation.

**Telehealth and Specialized Apparatuses:**

Telehealth arrangements assume a vital part in RPM, working with virtual counsels among patients and medical care suppliers. Video calls, secure informing, and other specialized instruments empower constant connections, permitting medical services experts to remotely survey patients' circumstances, give direction, and change therapy plans on a case by case basis.

**Information Investigation and Man-made reasoning (computer based intelligence):**

The sheer volume of information produced by RPM requires progressed examination and, at times, man-made intelligence applications to determine significant experiences. Information examination assist with distinguishing examples, patterns, and irregularities in persistent information, empowering medical services suppliers to settle on informed choices. Simulated intelligence calculations can add to prescient examination, risk definition, and customized care plans in light of individual patient information.

**Patient Entrances and Applications:**

Patient commitment is a basic part of RPM, and patient entrances or portable applications act as points of interaction for people to get to their wellbeing information, get instructive assets, and speak with medical care suppliers. Enabling patients with simple admittance to their wellbeing data cultivates a feeling of responsibility and joint effort in the administration of their circumstances.

3. **Uses of Far off Quiet Observing:**

**Ongoing Sickness The executives:**

RPM has demonstrated especially effective in the administration of ongoing illnesses like diabetes, hypertension, and cardiovascular breakdown. Consistent checking of essential signs and significant biomarkers permits medical care suppliers to mediate expeditiously because of vacillations in patients' wellbeing status. For people with persistent circumstances, RPM offers a proactive way to deal with care, decreasing the requirement for successive in-person visits while improving by and large sickness the board.

**Postoperative Consideration and Restoration:**

Following surgeries, RPM empowers medical services suppliers to remotely screen patients' recuperation. Wearable gadgets can follow portability, action levels, and important bodily functions, giving bits of knowledge into the post-operative recuperating process. This considers early identification of intricacies as well as works with customized restoration plans, advancing recuperation and diminishing the weight on the two patients and medical services offices.

**Maternal and Newborn child Wellbeing:**

RPM stretches out its advantages to maternal and baby wellbeing by permitting medical services suppliers to screen eager moms and infants from a distance. Wearable gadgets and associated sensors can follow maternal indispensable signs, fetal pulse, and baby development boundaries. This application is especially important for high-risk pregnancies and post pregnancy care, empowering convenient intercessions and upgrading the general prosperity of both mother and youngster.

**Maturing Populace and Home Medical care:**

As populaces age, the interest for locally established medical care arrangements increments. RPM gives a way to screen the wellbeing of the older in their homes, assisting medical services suppliers with distinguishing early indications of weakening or likely crises. This application upholds maturing set up, permitting people to keep up with their autonomy while getting proactive medical care administrations.

**Emotional well-being Observing:**

RPM is extending its degree to incorporate emotional well-being observing. Wearable gadgets and versatile applications can follow signs of mental prosperity, for example, rest designs, action levels, and feelings of anxiety. This all encompassing methodology perceives the interconnectedness of physical and psychological wellness, offering significant bits of knowledge for the administration of conditions like nervousness and sorrow.

4. **Advantages of Far off Tolerant Observing:**

**Early Discovery of Medical problems:**

One of the essential benefits of RPM is its capacity to work with early recognition of medical problems. Persistent observing permits medical care suppliers to recognize deviations from benchmark wellbeing measurements continuously, empowering opportune mediations. This proactive methodology can forestall the movement of conditions and lessen the probability of crisis hospitalizations.

**Further developed Ongoing Infection The executives:**

RPM fundamentally works on the administration of persistent sicknesses by giving a nonstop stream of information for medical care suppliers to survey. This approach takes into consideration customized care plans, acclimations to prescriptions, and way of life proposals in light of genuine world, everyday information. Patients with constant circumstances experience improved help and are better prepared to deal with their wellbeing.

**Diminished Medical services Expenses:**

By moving parts of medical services conveyance from customary settings to remote checking, RPM can possibly lessen medical services costs. Less medical clinic confirmations, diminished trauma center visits, and enhanced utilization of medical services assets add to cost investment funds. Also, early mediation and preventive measures can forestall the heightening of medical problems, further lessening generally medical care consumptions.

**Upgraded Patient Commitment and Strengthening:**

RPM enables patients to effectively take part in their medical services venture. The openness of continuous wellbeing information through persistent gateways or portable applications encourages a feeling of responsibility and commitment. Patients become accomplices in their consideration, settling on informed choices, sticking to treatment plans, and successfully dealing with their circumstances fully backed by medical care suppliers.

**Upgraded Asset Assignment:**

Remote observing empowers medical services suppliers to proficiently dispense assets more. By focusing on patients in light of their constant wellbeing status and mediation needs, suppliers can advance their work processes. This designated approach guarantees that assets are coordinated where they are most required, further developing generally medical services framework effectiveness.

**Customized and Information Driven Care:**

The abundance of information created by RPM works with customized and information driven care. Medical services suppliers can tailor mediations and care plans in view of individual patient profiles, changing systems in light of developing wellbeing patterns. This degree of personalization adds to more powerful and patient-driven medical care conveyance.

5. **Difficulties and Contemplations in Far off Quiet Checking:**

**Innovation Availability and Education:**

The far and wide reception of RPM faces difficulties connected with innovation openness and proficiency. Not all patients approach cell phones or wearable gadgets, and differences in advanced education might block viable use. Addressing these difficulties expects endeavors to upgrade innovation access, give training, and guarantee inclusivity in the organization of RPM arrangements.

**Information Security and Protection Concerns:**

The assortment, transmission, and capacity of touchy wellbeing information in RPM raise critical worries in regards to information security and protection. Guaranteeing consistence with administrative structures, executing powerful encryption gauges, and laying out clear rules for information taking care of are fundamental for fabricate trust among patients and medical services suppliers.

**Coordination with Existing Medical services Frameworks:**

Consistent coordination of RPM information with existing medical services frameworks, including EHRs, is pivotal for its viability. Fragmented joining might prompt disconnected care, information storehouses, and difficulties in getting to complete patient data. Accomplishing interoperability requires deliberate endeavors to lay out normalized information arrangements and correspondence conventions.

**Repayment and Monetary Models:**

The ongoing medical care repayment models frequently don't enough record for the worth conveyed by RPM. Moving to a repayment structure that perceives the advantages of remote observing represents a test. Laying out clear monetary models that boost medical services suppliers to take on and support RPM drives is fundamental for boundless reception.

**Client Adherence and Commitment:**

The outcome of RPM depends on client adherence and commitment. Guaranteeing that patients reliably utilize wearable gadgets, stick to observing conventions, and effectively draw in with telehealth stages is a relentless test. Planning easy to understand interfaces, giving training, and consolidating patient input are methodologies to upgrade client adherence.

**Administrative Consistence:**

Consistence with administrative prerequisites and norms is a basic thought in the organization of RPM arrangements. Complying with rules connected with information insurance, medical services practices, and innovation norms is fundamental for legitimate and moral reasons. Exploring the complex administrative scene requires an intensive comprehension of territorial and global medical services guidelines.

**Framework and Availability:**

The adequacy of RPM is dependent upon powerful computerized foundation and network. In districts with restricted admittance to rapid web or regions with deficient computerized framework, conveying RPM arrangements becomes testing. Addressing framework holes is essential to guarantee evenhanded admittance to remote observing capacities.

6. **Future Possibilities of Far off Understanding Checking:**

**Coordination of Cutting edge Sensors and Advances:**

The fate of RPM includes the combination of cutting edge sensors and innovations to widen the extent of observed boundaries. Wearables with improved sensor capacities, including biomarker recognition, ecological checking, and high level imaging, will give a more complete perspective on patients' wellbeing. Scaling down and expanded sensor awareness will add to the advancement of cutting edge RPM gadgets.

**Man-made brainpower for Prescient Examination:**

The mix of man-made brainpower for prescient examination holds huge expected in RPM. Computer based intelligence calculations can examine huge datasets to recognize designs, anticipate wellbeing patterns, and define patient dangers. This prescient ability upgrades the proactive administration of ailments, permitting medical services suppliers to intercede before issues heighten.

**Extension of Psychological wellness Observing:**

Psychological well-being observing inside the domain of RPM is ready for critical development. Wearable gadgets and advanced stages will progressively zero in on following mental prosperity pointers, for example, feelings of anxiety, rest examples, and mind-set varieties. This all encompassing methodology recognizes the interconnected idea of physical and psychological well-being, cultivating a more exhaustive comprehension of patients' general prosperity.

**Telehealth Reconciliation and Virtual Consideration Models:**

The reconciliation of RPM with telehealth stages and the development of virtual consideration models are fundamental to the fate of medical care conveyance. RPM will flawlessly coordinate with telehealth visits, giving continuous information during virtual conferences. Virtual consideration models will stretch out past wordy connections, consolidating constant remote observing as a standard part of care conveyance.

**Blockchain for Information Security:**

Blockchain innovation might assume a part in upgrading the security and respectability of RPM information. Decentralized and secure information stockpiling, combined with blockchain's abilities in guaranteeing information changelessness, could address concerns connected with information security and protection. This innovation can possibly upgrade trust in RPM frameworks, particularly in delicate medical care settings.

**Administrative Systems and Repayment Models:**

The development of administrative structures and repayment models is basic for the supported development of RPM. Clear rules that address the one of a kind parts of remote checking, combined with repayment structures that perceive the worth of RPM in working on understanding results and diminishing medical services costs, will urge medical services suppliers to embrace and put resources into these advances.

**Worldwide Openness and Value:**

Endeavors to improve the worldwide openness and value of RPM will be key to its future possibilities. Tending to differences in innovation access, computerized proficiency, and medical care foundation will guarantee that the advantages of RPM are acknowledged across assorted populaces and geological districts. Worldwide coordinated efforts and drives are fundamental to make comprehensive and impartial medical services arrangements.

**3.1 Examination of remote patient monitoring technologies**

The assessment of Distant Patient Checking (RPM) advances uncovers a unique scene portrayed by development, mix of cutting edge sensors, and a shift towards patient-driven care. As medical care develops, RPM innovations assume an essential part in expanding the scope of medical services past conventional settings, offering nonstop checking, information driven experiences, and customized mediations. This investigation digs into the assorted scope of RPM innovations, their applications, advantages, challenges, and the advancing fate of distant patient checking.

1. **Wearable Gadgets and Sensors:**
   Wearable gadgets furnished with cutting edge sensors structure the foundation of far off quiet checking advancements. These gadgets, going from smart-watches to clinical grade wearables, are intended to catch a heap of physiological information. Key imperative signs, for example, pulse, circulatory strain, oxygen immersion, and movement levels can be ceaselessly observed, giving an ongoing stream of wellbeing data. The development of wearable sensors has seen the incorporation of refined innovations, including photoplethysmography (PPG), accelerometers, and whirligigs, empowering exact and non-meddlesome infor-mation assortment.

   These wearables act as information gatherers as well as proposition a consistent and inconspicuous experience for patients. The comfort of wearable gadgets urges long haul adherence to observing conventions, vital for the adequacy of distant patient checking. Besides, wearables are progressively planned with easy to use interfaces, guaranteeing openness for people of different ages and innova-tive proficiency levels.

2. **Remote Observing Stages:**
   At the center of distant patient observing innovations are the remote checking stages. These stages act as concentrated center points for gathering, putting away, and breaking down the huge measures of information produced by wearable gadgets. Reconciliation with Electronic Wellbeing Records (EHRs) and other medical care frameworks guarantees that the information flawlessly streams into the more extensive medical care foundation. This reconciliation is fundamental for giving medical care experts a thorough perspective on patients' wellbeing status, taking into consideration informed independent direction and customized intercessions.

   The heartiness of these stages lies in their capacity to deal with assorted informa-tion types, going from essential signs and biomarkers to patient-revealed results. Furthermore, they frequently consolidate information examination capacities, empowering the distinguishing proof of examples, patterns, and oddities in persistent information. The incorporation of man-made brainpower further improves the scientific capacities, adding to prescient examination and custom-ized care suggestions.

3. **Telehealth and Specialized Apparatuses:**
   Telehealth arrangements and specialized apparatuses are fundamental parts of RPM advances, working with virtual communications between medical services suppliers and patients. Video calls, secure informing, and virtual visits consider constant correspondence, empowering medical care experts to survey patients' circumstances from a distance. These devices overcome any barrier between

in-person visits, offering a nonstop and open channel for medical services conveyance.

The incorporation of telehealth with RPM innovations is changing the idea of medical care meetings. During virtual visits, medical care suppliers can use the ongoing information gathered by wearable gadgets to illuminate their appraisals. This collaboration among telehealth and remote observing upgrades the proficiency of medical care conveyance, diminishes the requirement for superfluous in-person visits, and works with opportune mediations in view of dynamic wellbeing information.

4. **Information Investigation and Man-made consciousness (simulated intelligence):**

The sheer volume of information produced by RPM innovations requires progressed examination and computerized reasoning applications. Information examination devices assume a pivotal part in removing significant experiences from the constant stream of patient information. These experiences range from distinguishing unpretentious changes in essential signs to perceiving designs demonstrative of wellbeing patterns or likely issues.

Man-made consciousness applications, including AI calculations, add to prescient examination and customized care. By breaking down verifiable patient information, man-made intelligence can recognize risk factors, anticipate wellbeing directions, and suggest customized mediations. The combination of man-made intelligence improves the exactness of information examination as well as supports medical services experts in going with proactive and information driven choices.

5. **Patient Entrances and Versatile Applications:**

Patient commitment is a foundation of powerful far off persistent checking, and patient entryways or versatile applications act as the connection point through which people communicate with their wellbeing information. These stages give patients admittance to their ongoing wellbeing data, including crucial signs, drifts, and customized care plans. Patient entrances additionally act as instructive devices, offering assets and data to upgrade wellbeing proficiency.

The easy to use plan of these gateways and applications is fundamental for advancing dynamic patient interest. Clear perceptions of wellbeing information, instinctive route, and highlights that support correspondence with medical care suppliers add to a positive client experience. Engaging patients with simple admittance to their wellbeing data cultivates a feeling of pride and urges them to assume a functioning part in their consideration.

**Uses of Far off Quiet Observing Advancements:**

**Persistent Infection The board:**

RPM advancements have tracked down broad applications in the administration of constant sicknesses.

Persistent checking of imperative signs and important biomarkers permits medical care suppliers to follow the movement of conditions like diabetes, hypertension, and cardiovascular breakdown. Customized care plans can be contrived in view of genuine world, everyday information, enhancing illness the executives and decreasing the requirement for regular in-person visits.

**Postoperative Consideration and Restoration:**

Following surgeries, RPM advances add to postoperative consideration and recovery. Wearable gadgets can screen portability, action levels, and important bodily functions, giving bits of knowledge into the recuperation interaction. This application works with early identification of confusions as well as considers customized restoration plans, further developing by and large recuperation results.

**Maternal and Newborn child Wellbeing:**

RPM advances assume a critical part in maternal and baby wellbeing by empowering remote observing of hopeful moms and infants. Wearable gadgets and associated sensors can follow maternal indispensable signs, fetal pulse, and newborn child development boundaries. This application is especially important for high-risk pregnancies and post pregnancy care, improving the general prosperity of both mother and kid.

**Maturing Populace and Home Medical services:**

As the worldwide populace ages, RPM advancements support locally established medical services arrangements. Remote observing permits medical services suppliers to follow the wellbeing of the older in their homes, empowering early discovery of medical problems or crises. This application upholds maturing set up, permitting people to keep up with their freedom while getting proactive medical care administrations.

**Psychological wellness Observing:**

RPM advances are growing their extension to incorporate emotional well-being observing. Wearable gadgets and portable applications can follow marks of mental prosperity, for example, rest designs, movement levels, and feelings of anxiety. This all encompassing methodology perceives the interconnectedness of physical and psychological wellness, giving significant experiences to the administration of conditions like nervousness and wretchedness.

**Advantages of Distant Patient Observing Innovations:**

**Early Recognition of Medical problems:**

The constant observing given by RPM innovations works with the early location of medical problems. Constant information streams empower medical services suppliers to speedily distinguish deviations from benchmark wellbeing measurements. This proactive methodology can forestall the movement of conditions and decrease the probability of crisis hospitalizations.

**Further developed Persistent Infection The board:**

RPM advances fundamentally upgrade the administration of persistent illnesses. Nonstop information streams consider customized care plans, acclimations to prescriptions, and way of life suggestions in light of genuine world, everyday information. Patients with constant circumstances experience improved help and are better prepared to deal with their wellbeing.

**Diminished Medical care Expenses:**

By moving parts of medical services conveyance from conventional settings to remote checking, RPM advances can possibly decrease medical care costs. Less medical clinic affirmations, diminished trauma center visits, and upgraded utilization of medical services assets add to cost investment funds. Moreover, early intercession and preventive measures can forestall the acceleration of medical problems, further lessening in general medical care consumptions.

**Upgraded Patient Commitment and Strengthening:**

RPM advancements engage patients to effectively take part in their medical services venture. Admittance to ongoing wellbeing information encourages a feeling of pride and commitment. Patients become accomplices in their consideration, settling on informed choices, sticking to treatment plans, and successfully dealing with their circumstances fully backed by medical services suppliers.

**Streamlined Asset Designation:**

Remote observing advances empower medical services suppliers to proficiently designate assets more. By focusing on patients in view of their constant wellbeing status and mediation needs, suppliers can advance their work processes. This designated approach guarantees that assets are coordinated where they are most required, further developing in general medical services framework effectiveness.

**Customized and Information Driven Care:**

The abundance of information produced by RPM advances works with customized and information driven care. Medical services suppliers can tailor mediations and care plans in light of individual patient profiles, changing procedures because of advancing wellbeing patterns. This degree of personalization adds to more powerful and patient-driven medical services conveyance.

**Difficulties and Contemplations in Far off Tolerant Checking Advancements:**

**Innovation Openness and Education:**

The reception of RPM advances faces difficulties connected with innovation openness and proficiency. Not all patients approach cell phones or wearable gadgets, and abberations in computerized proficiency might thwart successful use.

Addressing these difficulties expects endeavors to upgrade innovation access, give training, and guarantee inclusivity in the arrangement of RPM arrangements.

**Information Security and Protection Concerns:**

The delicate idea of wellbeing information in RPM advancements raises critical worries in regards to information security and protection. Guaranteeing consistence with administrative systems, executing vigorous encryption gauges, and laying out clear rules for information taking care of are crucial for fabricate trust among patients and medical services suppliers.

**Incorporation with Existing Medical care Frameworks:**

Consistent incorporation of RPM information with existing medical care frameworks, including EHRs, is urgent for its viability. Fragmented mix might prompt disconnected care, information storehouses, and difficulties in getting to complete patient data. Accomplishing interoperability requires purposeful endeavors to lay out normalized information configurations and correspondence conventions.

**Repayment and Monetary Models:**

The ongoing medical care repayment models frequently don't satisfactorily represent the worth conveyed by RPM advances. Moving to a repayment structure that perceives the advantages of remote observing represents a test. Laying out clear monetary models that boost medical care suppliers to embrace and support RPM drives is fundamental for far reaching reception.

**Client Adherence and Commitment:**

The progress of RPM advancements depends on client adherence and commitment. Guaranteeing that patients reliably utilize wearable gadgets, stick to checking conventions, and effectively draw in with telehealth stages is a persevering test. Planning easy to use interfaces, giving instruction, and integrating patient criticism are methodologies to upgrade client adherence.

**Administrative Consistence:**

Consistence with administrative necessities and norms is a basic thought in the sending of RPM innovations. Complying with rules connected with information security, medical services practices, and innovation guidelines is fundamental for lawful and moral reasons. Exploring the complex administrative scene requires a careful comprehension of territorial and worldwide medical services guidelines.

**Foundation and Availability:**

The viability of RPM advances is dependent upon strong computerized framework and network. In locales with restricted admittance to rapid web or regions with lacking advanced framework, conveying RPM arrangements becomes testing. Addressing foundation holes is vital to guarantee fair admittance to remote observing abilities.

**Future Possibilities of Far off Persistent Checking Advances:**

**Incorporation of Cutting edge Sensors and Advances:**

The eventual fate of RPM innovations includes the incorporation of cutting edge sensors and advancements to widen the extent of observed boundaries. Wearables with upgraded sensor capacities, including biomarker discovery, ecological observing, and high level imaging, will give a more far reaching perspective on patients' wellbeing. Scaling down and expanded sensor responsiveness will add to the improvement of cutting edge RPM gadgets.

**Man-made brainpower for Prescient Investigation:**

The mix of man-made reasoning for prescient examination holds colossal likely in RPM. Simulated intelligence calculations can break down tremendous datasets to distinguish designs, foresee wellbeing patterns, and separate patient dangers. This prescient capacity upgrades the proactive administration of ailments, permitting medical care suppliers to mediate before issues heighten.

**Extension of Psychological wellness Checking:**

RPM advances are ready for critical extension in psychological well-being checking. Wearable gadgets and advanced stages will progressively zero in on following mental prosperity pointers, for example, feelings of anxiety, rest examples, and temperament varieties. This comprehensive methodology recognizes the interconnected idea of physical and emotional well-being, giving significant bits of knowledge to the administration of conditions like uneasiness and sadness.

**Telehealth Joining and Virtual Consideration Models:**

The combination of RPM advancements with telehealth stages and the development of virtual consideration models are vital to the fate of medical services conveyance. RPM will consistently coordinate with telehealth visits, giving constant information during virtual meetings. Virtual consideration models will reach out past wordy cooperations, consolidating persistent remote checking as a standard part of care conveyance.

**Blockchain for Information Security:**

Blockchain innovation might assume a part in improving the security and honesty of RPM information. Decentralized and secure information stockpiling, combined with blockchain's abilities in guaranteeing information permanence, could address concerns connected with information security and protection. This innovation can possibly upgrade trust in RPM frameworks, particularly in touchy medical services settings.

**Administrative Structures and Repayment Models:**

The advancement of administrative structures and repayment models is basic for the supported development of RPM innovations.

Clear rules that address the special parts of remote checking, combined with repayment structures that perceive the worth of RPM in working on understanding results and decreasing medical services costs, will urge medical services suppliers to embrace and put resources into these advances.

**Worldwide Availability and Value:**

Endeavors to upgrade the worldwide openness and value of RPM innovations will be fundamental to their future possibilities. Tending to differences in innovation access, computerized education, and medical care framework will guarantee that the advantages of RPM are acknowledged across assorted populaces and geological locales. Worldwide joint efforts and drives are fundamental to make comprehensive and impartial medical care arrangements.

**3.2 Use cases in chronic disease management and postoperative care**

Far off Quiet Observing (RPM) advances have introduced another period of medical services conveyance, and their effect is especially articulated in the administration of constant illnesses and postoperative consideration. This segment investigates the extraordinary use instances of RPM advancements in these basic spaces, revealing insight into the manners by which persistent observing, information driven bits of knowledge, and customized mediations add to worked on quiet results and upgraded medical care proficiency.

**Persistent Illness The executives:**

**RPM in Diabetes The executives:**

Constant infections, for example, diabetes, benefit altogether from RPM advances. Ceaseless checking of blood glucose levels through wearable gadgets gives constant information, empowering medical services suppliers to follow changes and patterns. This powerful way to deal with diabetes the board takes into consideration customized acclimations to prescription regimens and way of life suggestions. Patients, furnished with noteworthy bits of knowledge and criticism, can effectively partake in dealing with their condition, prompting better glycemic control and diminishing the gamble of complexities.

**RPM in Hypertension The executives:**

Hypertension, one more common persistent condition, is successfully tended to through distant patient observing. Wearable gadgets furnished with pulse sensors consider ceaseless checking of circulatory strain varieties.

Medical care suppliers can recognize examples and patterns, changing medicine measurements and way of life suggestions as needs be. By mediating progressively, RPM advances add to ideal circulatory strain control, decreasing the gamble of cardiovascular occasions and upgrading the general personal satisfaction for people with hypertension.

**RPM in Cardiovascular breakdown The executives:**

Cardiovascular breakdown, a complex constant condition, presents huge difficulties in administration. RPM advances assume a vital part in giving complete consideration to people with cardiovascular breakdown. Wearable gadgets can screen imperative signs, for example, pulse, respiratory rate, and oxygen immersion, offering an all encompassing perspective on a patient's cardiovascular wellbeing. The nonstop stream of information empowers early location of changes in the patient's condition, working with ideal mediations to forestall intensifications and hospitalizations. This proactive methodology works on tolerant results as well as decreases the weight on medical services assets.

**RPM in Respiratory Circumstances:**

Respiratory circumstances, including constant obstructive aspiratory sickness (COPD) and asthma, track down viable help in RPM advancements. Wearable gadgets and associated sensors can screen respiratory rates, lung capability, and oxygen levels. By ceaselessly following these boundaries, medical care suppliers can distinguish patterns characteristic of deteriorating respiratory capability. This considers early mediation, customized changes in accordance with prescription plans, and distant direction on overseeing intensifications. Patients with respiratory circumstances experience further developed side effect control and a superior personal satisfaction through the proactive utilization of RPM innovations.

**Postoperative Consideration:**

### RPM in Muscular Medical procedure Recuperation:

Postoperative consideration is a basic stage in the medical services excursion, and RPM advancements contribute essentially to the recuperation cycle, particularly in muscular medical procedure. Wearable gadgets can screen versatility, joint scope of movement, and important bodily functions, giving bits of knowledge into the patient's recuperation progress. This consistent observing permits medical care suppliers to identify complexities or deviations from the normal recuperation direction almost immediately. By remotely surveying the patient's condition, medical care experts can tailor restoration plans, suggest works out, and give direction, enhancing the postoperative recuperation experience.

### RPM in Cardiovascular Medical procedure Recuperation:

Heart medical procedure, whether coronary course sidestep uniting or valve substitution, requires cautious postoperative observing.

RPM innovations assume a critical part in remotely following crucial signs, for example, pulse and mood, circulatory strain, and oxygen immersion. Constant checking gives experiences into the cardiovascular recuperation process, permitting medical services suppliers to recognize likely complexities, like arrhythmias or changes in hemodynamic security. Convenient intercessions in light of constant information add to a smoother postoperative recuperation and a decreased gamble of confusions.

### RPM in Gastrointestinal Medical procedure Recuperation:

Gastrointestinal medical procedures, including techniques, for example, laparoscopic medical procedures or colorectal medical procedures, benefit from the persistent checking empowered by RPM innovations. Wearable gadgets can follow boundaries, for example, stomach development, pulse, and postoperative torment levels. This ongoing information permits medical services suppliers to remotely survey the patient's recuperation, distinguish issues like careful site diseases or unreasonable agony, and intercede appropriately. The customized bits of knowledge from RPM add to a more persistent driven and effective postoperative consideration model.

### RPM in Bariatric Medical procedure Recuperation:

Bariatric medical procedures for weight the executives frequently require cautious postoperative checking. RPM innovations offer an answer by giving constant experiences into fundamental signs, movement levels, and wholesome markers. This checking permits medical services suppliers to evaluate the viability of weight reduction intercessions, recognize potential difficulties like supplement inadequacies, and proposition customized direction on dietary and way of life changes. The distant idea of RPM in bariatric medical procedure recuperation advances patient comfort and adherence to postoperative consideration plans.

### Advantages and Difficulties:

### Advantages of RPM in Constant Sickness The board:

The utilization instances of RPM in constant sickness the executives offer a few advantages. Above all else is the capacity to identify changes in wellbeing status progressively, empowering early mediations and forestalling the movement of constant circumstances. Customized care plans, informed by ceaseless checking, lead to further developed sickness the executives and streamlined therapy regimens. Patients, enabled with constant bits of knowledge and progressing support, experience improved commitment and better adherence to their consideration plans. Also, the decrease in crisis hospitalizations and medical services costs adds to the general proficiency of medical services conveyance.

**Advantages of RPM in Postoperative Consideration:**

RPM advances in postoperative consideration achieve groundbreaking advantages. Ceaseless observing takes into consideration early identification of confusions, limiting the gamble of unfavorable occasions and working on understanding security. Customized recuperation plans, in view of ongoing information, add to upgraded restoration and a more custom-made postoperative experience. Patients, upheld by RPM, frequently experience decreased postoperative pressure, improved comfort, and a feeling of network with their medical care suppliers. Moreover, the smoothed out way to deal with postoperative consideration adds to asset improvement inside medical care frameworks.

**Challenges in Ongoing Illness The board with RPM:**

Regardless of the apparent advantages, the execution of RPM in persistent sickness the executives accompanies its arrangement of difficulties. Innovation openness and computerized education among patients can affect the broad reception of RPM arrangements. Information security and security concerns require strong measures to guarantee the assurance of delicate wellbeing data. Incorporating RPM information consistently with existing medical care frameworks and beating repayment challenges are diligent obstacles. Additionally, supporting client adherence over the long haul and resolving issues connected with administrative consistence present continuous difficulties in the execution of RPM in ongoing sickness the board.

**Challenges in Postoperative Consideration with RPM:**

In postoperative consideration, challenges related with RPM incorporate guaranteeing patient adherence to wearable gadgets and observing conventions. Addressing concerns connected with information security and protection is vital, particularly with regards to delicate postoperative wellbeing data. The mix of RPM information into existing postoperative consideration work processes requires consistent interoperability with electronic wellbeing records. Conquering repayment models that may not completely represent the worth of remote checking in postoperative consideration is a continuous test. Moreover, the requirement for powerful persistent training and backing to improve the client experience stays a basic part of effective RPM execution in postoperative consideration.

**3.3 Discussion on how remote monitoring enhances patient engagement and reduces healthcare costs**

Distant Patient Observing (RPM) remains at the bleeding edge of groundbreaking medical services innovations, offering a powerful way to deal with patient consideration. This conversation dives into the significant job of remote checking in upgrading patient commitment and simultaneously diminishing medical services costs.

As innovation develops, the collaboration between quiet driven care and cost-proficiency turns out to be progressively obvious, situating RPM as a critical driver of advancement in the medical services scene.

**Upgrading Patient Commitment:**

Patient commitment is a foundation of powerful medical care, and RPM innovations assume an essential part in cultivating dynamic cooperation. Through the organization of wearable gadgets, associated sensors, and telehealth stages, RPM carries medical services into the day to day routines of patients, making a nonstop criticism circle among people and their medical services suppliers.

One of the essential ways RPM upgrades patient commitment is by giving continuous admittance to wellbeing information. Wearable gadgets outfitted with sensors consistently screen imperative signs, action levels, and other pertinent measurements. Patients can get to this data through easy to understand interfaces, frequently as versatile applications or patient entries. This availability enables people to follow their wellbeing status, grasp designs, and effectively take part in the administration of persistent circumstances.

Moreover, RPM works with proactive correspondence among patients and medical services suppliers. Telehealth stages empower virtual conferences, permitting people to associate with their medical services group from a distance. During these virtual visits, medical care suppliers can use the ongoing information gathered by RPM gadgets to illuminate their evaluations. This cooperative methodology cultivates a feeling of organization among patients and suppliers, where shared independent direction turns into a focal precept of medical services conveyance.

The instructive part of RPM likewise adds to upgraded patient commitment. Patient entrances and versatile applications frequently incorporate assets, instructive materials, and customized care plans. By giving data customized to individual wellbeing profiles, RPM engages patients with information, cultivating wellbeing proficiency and empowering them to arrive at informed conclusions about their consideration. This schooling driven commitment prompts more noteworthy adherence to treatment plans, drug regimens, and way of life adjustments.

**Lessening Medical care Expenses:**

Simultaneously, the execution of RPM advancements can possibly essentially decrease medical care costs. The expense viability originates from different components that improve asset use, forestall exorbitant intricacies, and smooth out medical services conveyance.

One of the essential expense saving parts of RPM is the decrease in emergency clinic confirmations. Constant observing empowers the early identification of changes in patients' wellbeing status, permitting medical services suppliers to mediate before conditions raise with the eventual result of requiring hospitalization.

This proactive methodology is especially helpful for people with ongoing circumstances, where convenient intercessions can forestall intensifications and the related significant expenses of crisis clinic visits.

Trauma center visits, frequently an exorbitant part of medical services, can be moderated through RPM. By engaging patients to effectively deal with their wellbeing and giving convenient mediations, RPM limits the requirement for dire consideration. The availability of virtual meetings through telehealth stages further decreases the dependence on crisis administrations for non-emanant circumstances. This redirection of medical services use saves costs as well as enhances the utilization of medical services assets.

Besides, RPM adds to the enhancement of medical care work processes. By focusing on patients in view of constant wellbeing status and mediation needs, medical care suppliers can distribute assets all the more productively. This designated approach guarantees that medical care experts center their endeavors where they are generally required, lessening pointless methods, tests, and intercessions. The smoothed out work process adds to further developed generally medical services framework productivity and asset portion.

The avoidance of difficulties is one more road through which RPM lessens medical care costs. For constant circumstances like diabetes, cardiovascular breakdown, and hypertension, early location of deviations from benchmark wellbeing measurements takes into account opportune changes in accordance with treatment plans. This proactive administration forestalls the movement of conditions, lessening the requirement for costly medicines, hospitalizations, and broad intercessions.

The monetary effect of RPM is additionally stressed by the shift from responsive to proactive medical care. Customary models of care frequently include tending to medical problems after they have showed, prompting greater expenses related with cutting edge therapies and crisis care. Conversely, RPM works with a proactive methodology by persistently observing wellbeing boundaries and empowering early intercessions. This shift lessens the financial weight related with treating progressed stage infections and intricacies.

**Difficulties and Contemplations:**

While the expected advantages of remote observing in improving patient commitment and decreasing medical care costs are significant, difficulties and contemplations should be tended to for broad reception. Innovation openness and computerized education among different patient populaces stay a huge obstacle. Endeavors are expected to guarantee evenhanded admittance to RPM arrangements, considering financial factors and differing levels of mechanical education.

Information security and protection concerns represent another test. The delicate idea of wellbeing information requires strong measures to defend patient data. Consistence with administrative systems, execution of encryption measures, and straightforward correspondence about information taking care of practices are crucial for fabricate trust among patients and medical services suppliers.

The reconciliation of RPM information with existing medical services frameworks, including Electronic Wellbeing Records (EHRs), is basic for its adequacy. Fragmented coordination might prompt disconnected care, information storehouses, and difficulties in getting to thorough patient data. Accomplishing interoperability requires normalized information organizations and correspondence conventions, requiring co-operative endeavors inside the medical care biological system.

Repayment models present a critical thought in the reception of RPM. The on-going medical services repayment designs may not completely represent the worth conveyed by remote observing. Moving to a repayment model that perceives the advantages of RPM represents a test, and clear monetary models boosting medical care suppliers to take on and support RPM drives are fundamental.

Client adherence and commitment are diligent difficulties. Guaranteeing that patients reliably utilize wearable gadgets, stick to checking conventions, and effectively draw in with telehealth stages requires continuous endeavors. Planning easy to understand interfaces, giving instruction, and integrating patient input are systems to improve client adherence and, thusly, the outcome of RPM executions.

**3.4 Ethical considerations and challenges in implementing remote patient monitoring systems**

The execution of Distant Patient Observing (RPM) frameworks presents a horde of moral contemplations and difficulties that request cautious route. While RPM holds the commitment of upgrading medical services conveyance and patient results, it likewise brings to the cutting edge complex issues connected with protection, infor-mation security, patient independence, and the evenhanded admittance to innovation. This conversation investigates the moral scene encompassing RPM, revealing insight into the difficulties that should be addressed to guarantee mindful and patient-driven arrangement of these groundbreaking innovations.

1. **Protection and Information Security:**

   Protection is a basic moral guideline in medical care, and RPM frameworks intrinsically include the assortment and transmission of delicate wellbeing in-formation. The consistent checking of fundamental signs, patient ways of be-having, and other wellbeing measurements raises worries about the classification and security of this data. Guaranteeing that patient information is shielded from unapproved access, breaks, or abuse is a fundamental moral obligation.

   Challenges emerge in characterizing and executing strong information safety efforts. Encryption conventions, secure transmission channels, and tough access controls are fundamental parts of protecting patient data. Also, RPM frame-works should comply to administrative systems, for example, the Medical cover-age Conveyability and Responsibility Act (HIPAA) in the US or the Overall Information Assurance Guideline (GDPR) in the European Association to guarantee legitimate consistence and security of patient protection.

   Adjusting the basic of information security with the requirement for consistent data trade represents a continuous moral test. Finding some kind of harmony requires a nuanced approach that focuses on understanding protection while working with the successful utilization of wellbeing information for checking and intercession purposes.

2. **Informed Assent and Patient Independence:**

Regarding patient independence is a foundation of moral medical care rehearses. With regards to RPM, getting educated assent turns into a basic thought. Patients should be completely educated about the nature regarding remote checking, the sorts of information gathered, how the information will be utilized, and the likely ramifications for their consideration.

Challenges in getting educated assent come from the dynamic and constant nature of RPM. Not at all like conventional medical services intercessions where assent can be gotten before a particular technique, RPM includes progressing information assortment. This requires straightforward correspondence about the drawn out nature of observing and the possible changes in the checking boundaries over the long haul.

Moreover, guaranteeing that patients have the choice to select in or quit RPM support is urgent for maintaining their independence. Moral contemplations stretch out to addressing situations where patients might choose to end observing or deny their assent. Clear correspondence channels and available systems for quitting are fundamental parts of a morally solid RPM execution.

3. **Value and Access:**

The moral basic of giving fair admittance to medical services is emphasizd in the organization of RPM frameworks. Differences in admittance to innovation, computerized education, and financial elements can make imbalances in the capacity of people to profit from remote checking.

Guaranteeing that weak populaces, incorporating those with restricted admittance to cell phones, web network, or those dwelling in underserved regions, are not left behind is a huge moral test. The improvement of comprehensive systems that address these incongruities and elevate fair admittance to RPM innovations is fundamental for relieving wellbeing imbalances.

Also, the potential for intensifying existing medical services incongruities should be painstakingly thought of. In the event that specific populaces face obstructions to getting to RPM, there is a gamble of additional underestimation. Moral execution requires proactive measures to connect these holes, including local area commitment, training drives, and designated mediations to guarantee that the advantages of RPM are acknowledged across different socioeconomics.

4. **Straightforwardness and Trust:**

Laying out and keeping up with trust between medical services suppliers, innovation designers, and patients is central to the moral execution of RPM frameworks. Straightforwardness in correspondence with respect to the objectives, advantages, and expected dangers of remote checking is basic for building and supporting trust.

Challenges emerge in guaranteeing that patients have a reasonable comprehension of how their information will be utilized, who will approach it, and how it will impact their consideration. Furnishing patients with straightforward data about the calculations utilized for information examination, the safety efforts set up, and the expected ramifications of checking on their treatment plans encourages a feeling of organization and trust.

Addressing concerns connected with the likely abuse of wellbeing information by outsiders, for example, insurance agency or managers, is a moral objective. RPM executions should focus on the insurance of patient interests and classification, guaranteeing people that their wellbeing information will be utilized exclusively for the reasons for observing and further developing their medical care results.

5. **Clinical Legitimacy and Responsibility:**

The moral execution of RPM frameworks requires a powerful groundwork of clinical legitimacy. The exactness and unwavering quality of the information gathered by wearable gadgets and sensors influence the honesty of clinical choices in view of that data. Medical care suppliers bear a moral obligation to guarantee that the innovations utilized for remote observing are clinically approved and satisfy laid out guidelines.

Challenges emerge in the fast development of innovation and the rise of new gadgets. Guaranteeing that medical services suppliers are outfitted with the fundamental preparation and training to decipher and follow up on the information produced by RPM frameworks is a continuous test. The moral basic includes a promise to persistent learning, proof based practice, and normal reports on the clinical legitimacy of checking gadgets.

Responsibility is another pivotal moral thought. Laying out clear lines of liability regarding the understanding of RPM information, correspondence with patients, and dynamic in view of remote observing discoveries is fundamental. Moral systems should incorporate instruments for tending to blunders, breakdowns, or misinterpretations of information, with an emphasis on limiting possible mischief to patients.

# *Chapter 4*

## Smart Health Apps and Platforms

Shrewd wellbeing applications and stages have arisen as extraordinary devices in the domain of medical services, utilizing innovation to upgrade different parts of health, avoidance, conclusion, and therapy. This conversation investigates the scene of shrewd wellbeing applications and stages, analyzing their functionalities, advantages, challenges, and the general effect they have on the medical care biological system.

**Outline of Savvy Wellbeing Applications and Stages:**

Savvy wellbeing applications and stages address a different exhibit of computerized devices intended to help people in dealing with their wellbeing and prosperity. These advances influence the capacities of cell phones, wearables, and other associated gadgets to furnish clients with customized bits of knowledge, ongoing checking, and intelligent highlights that engage them to play a functioning job in their wellbeing.

**Functionalities:**

Shrewd wellbeing applications and stages offer many functionalities that take special care of various parts of medical services. These functionalities can incorporate wellbeing observing, medicine the executives, wellness following, telehealth administrations, psychological well-being support, and customized wellbeing proposals. Reconciliation with sensors and wearables considers the assortment of fundamental signs, action levels, rest designs, and other wellbeing related information.

**Benefits:**

The advantages of savvy wellbeing applications and stages are complex. One of the essential benefits is the democratization of medical services data and access. Clients can helpfully get to wellbeing related assets, screen their wellbeing measurements, and get convenient direction, regardless of their geological area. This democratization adds to preventive consideration, early discovery of medical problems, and further developed wellbeing results.

Personalization is another key advantage. Shrewd wellbeing applications influence information investigation and computerized reasoning to tailor suggestions and mediations in view of individual wellbeing profiles. This customized approach upgrades the adequacy of intercessions, prompting more significant and designated wellbeing enhancements.

Telehealth administrations implanted in shrewd wellbeing stages work with far off counsels, separating geological hindrances and growing admittance to medical services experts. This is especially huge in situations where in-person visits might be testing or unrealistic.

**Challenges:**

Regardless of the promising advantages, the execution of savvy wellbeing applications and stages isn't without challenges. Interoperability stays a huge obstacle, with different applications and gadgets working in storehouses, possibly prompting divided wellbeing records and deficient patient profiles. Accomplishing consistent mix between various stages and guaranteeing that wellbeing information can be shared across frameworks are progressing difficulties.

Information security and protection concerns are basic contemplations. The delicate idea of wellbeing data makes it an objective for digital dangers. Moral treatment of wellbeing information, adherence to protection guidelines, and strong safety efforts are basic to assemble and keep up with client trust.

The advanced separation presents difficulties connected with availability. Not all people have equivalent admittance to cell phones, wearables, or dependable web network. Addressing these differences is fundamental to forestall the intensification of existing medical services disparities.

**Preventive Wellbeing and Health Applications:**

**Wellbeing Checking:**

Preventive wellbeing and wellbeing applications frequently integrate wellbeing checking highlights that empower clients to follow different imperative signs and wellbeing measurements. These can incorporate pulse, circulatory strain, rest designs, actual work, and the sky is the limit from there. Wearable gadgets, for example, smartwatches and wellness trackers, assume a critical part in nonstop checking, furnishing clients with constant input on their wellbeing status.

These applications engage people to proactively deal with their wellbeing by distinguishing examples and patterns in their information. For instance, a wellness application might investigate action levels and give proposals to keeping a sound way of life, while a rest following application can offer bits of knowledge into rest quality and recommend upgrades.

**Sustenance and Wellness Following:**

Sustenance and wellness following applications are basic to preventive wellbeing methodologies. These applications permit clients to log their dietary admission, track calorie utilization, and screen healthful substance. Furthermore, wellness following highlights help people put forth and accomplish wellness objectives, screen exercise meetings, and get customized practice suggestions.

The gamification of wellness applications, where clients can acquire remunerates or rival companions, adds a component of commitment, spurring people to stick to their wellness schedules. These stages add to preventive wellbeing by advancing smart dieting propensities, normal active work, and generally prosperity.

**Psychological wellness and Stress The executives:**

Psychological well-being applications have acquired conspicuousness lately, tending to the developing consciousness of the significance of mental prosperity. These applications offer instruments for pressure the executives, care, contemplation, and mind-set following. Clients can get to directed contemplation meetings, unwinding activities, and assets for overseeing uneasiness and stress.

The reconciliation of psychological well-being highlights into shrewd wellbeing stages recognizes the all encompassing nature of prosperity. By giving devices to both physical and psychological well-being, these applications add to an exhaustive way to deal with preventive consideration.

**Symptomatic and Observing Applications:**

**Side effect Checkers:**

Indicative applications, frequently including side effect checkers, enable clients to evaluate their medical issue in light of detailed side effects. These applications use calculations to investigate client inputted side effects and give fundamental experiences into potential medical problems. While not a substitute for proficient clinical exhortation, these devices can help clients in settling on informed conclusions about looking for clinical consideration.

Challenges related with side effect checkers incorporate the requirement for exact information input, the potential for confusion of side effects, and the significance of underlining these devices as strong instead of demonstrative.

**Ongoing Sickness The board:**

Shrewd wellbeing applications assume an essential part in the administration of constant sicknesses. Patients with conditions like diabetes, hypertension, or cardio-vascular infections can utilize applications to screen their wellbeing boundaries, track drug adherence, and get customized care plans.

These applications empower medical care suppliers to remotely screen patients' circumstances and mediate continuously when deviations from gauge wellbeing measurements are identified. This proactive way to deal with constant illness the executives adds to worked on persistent results and diminished medical care costs related with preventable inconveniences.

**Drug The executives:**

Drug the executives applications help clients in coordinating and sticking to their prescription regimens. These applications frequently incorporate elements, for example, drug updates, dose following, and pill recognizable proof instruments. By advancing prescription adherence, these applications add to the compelling administration of ongoing circumstances and the anticipation of unfriendly occasions.

Challenges in prescription administration applications incorporate the requirement for precise drug input, thought of likely communications, and resolving issues connected with client carelessness or deliberate non-adherence.

**Telehealth Stages:**

Telehealth stages address a critical development in medical care conveyance, utilizing computerized innovation to work with far off meetings among patients and medical care suppliers. These stages frequently coordinate video conferencing, secure informing, and document sharing to empower virtual visits.

**Far off Conferences:**

Telehealth stages offer an answer for difficulties connected with geological hindrances and restricted admittance to medical care administrations. Patients can associate with medical care experts for standard check-ups, follow-up arrangements, or conferences without the requirement for in-person visits.

The accommodation of far off conferences is especially important in situations where patients face versatility challenges, live in far off regions, or require continuous observing for persistent circumstances. Telehealth stages add to further developed admittance to opportune medical care administrations, prompting more proactive and preventive consideration.

**E-remedies and Virtual Checking:**

Incorporated with electronic wellbeing records (EHRs) and brilliant wellbeing applications, telehealth stages work with the consistent sharing of patient data. Medical care suppliers can create e-solutions, request analytic tests, and screen patients' wellbeing information from a distance.

The virtual observing abilities of telehealth stages reach out past video conferences. By coordinating with wearables and brilliant wellbeing applications, these stages can get to continuous wellbeing measurements, empowering a more exhaustive comprehension of patients' wellbeing status.

**Difficulties and Contemplations:**

**Interoperability:**

Interoperability stays a tenacious test in the shrewd wellbeing application environment. Numerous applications and stages work freely, prompting divided wellbeing records and deficient patient profiles. Accomplishing consistent joining across various frameworks, including EHRs, wearables, and telehealth stages, is fundamental for giving a brought together and thorough perspective on persistent wellbeing.

**Information Security and Protection:**

Information security and protection concerns are vital in the domain of shrewd wellbeing applications and stages. The assortment, stockpiling, and transmission of delicate wellbeing information require powerful safety efforts to forestall unapproved access, information breaks, and digital dangers. Adherence to protection guidelines, like HIPAA and GDPR, is urgent for building and keeping up with client trust.

**Advanced Separation and Openness:**

The advanced separation presents difficulties connected with the openness of savvy wellbeing applications and stages. Not all people have equivalent admittance to cell phones, wearables, or dependable web network. Addressing these differences is fundamental to forestall the worsening of existing medical care imbalances.

Endeavors to connect the computerized partition incorporate drives to give reasonable gadgets, advance advanced education, and guarantee that shrewd wellbeing advances are planned in view of inclusivity.

**Client Commitment and Adherence:**

Client commitment and adherence are basic elements in the outcome of savvy wellbeing applications. Supporting client interest, guaranteeing steady utilization of observing gadgets, and elevating long haul adherence to wellbeing intercessions are progressing difficulties. Planning easy to use interfaces, consolidating gamification components, and giving customized criticism are methodologies to improve client commitment.

**Administrative Consistence:**

Administrative consistence is a perplexing scene in the quickly developing field of shrewd wellbeing applications. Guaranteeing that these advancements comply with local and worldwide guidelines, including information security regulations and clinical gadget guidelines, is fundamental. Engineers and suppliers should keep up to date with administrative updates and take part in straightforward correspondence in regards to consistence measures.

**Moral Contemplations:**

Moral contemplations in brilliant wellbeing applications envelop issues like informed assent, client independence, and the mindful utilization of wellbeing information. Clear correspondence about information utilization, straightforwardness in algorithmic direction, and client strengthening in controlling their wellbeing data are moral objectives. Tending to expected predispositions in calculations and guaranteeing that wellbeing mediations are proof based add to the moral arrangement of shrewd wellbeing advances.

**4.1 Overview of mobile applications designed for health and wellness**

The coming of portable applications has introduced an extraordinary time in the domain of wellbeing and health. These applications, generally alluded to as wellbeing and health applications, influence the capacities of cell phones to offer a different scope of functionalities pointed toward upgrading different parts of individual prosperity. This complete outline investigates the scene of portable applications intended for wellbeing and wellbeing, digging into their functionalities, advantages, challenges, and the general effect they have on the all encompassing soundness of clients.

**Functionalities of Wellbeing and Health Applications:**

Wellbeing and wellbeing applications envelop an expansive range of functionalities taking care of various components of individual wellbeing. These functionalities can be ordered into a few key regions, each adding to a complete way to deal with prosperity:

**Wellness Following:**

Wellness following applications are intended to screen and break down active work, furnishing clients with experiences into their work-out schedules, everyday advances, and generally wellness levels. These applications frequently coordinate with sensors in cell phones or wearable gadgets to gather information on advances taken, distance covered, calories consumed, and even pulse during proactive tasks. Clients can put forth wellness objectives, keep tabs on their development, and get continuous criticism on their exercises.

**Nourishment and Diet The executives:**

Sustenance applications help clients in dealing with their dietary propensities by offering highlights for feast arranging, calorie following, and nourishing examination. These applications might incorporate data sets of food things with nourishing data, empowering clients to log their dinners, screen their calorie admission, and settle on informed decisions about their eating routine. Some applications go past fundamental calorie counting and give customized proposals in light of clients' wellbeing objectives and dietary inclinations.

**Psychological well-being and Stress The board:**

Emotional well-being applications center around supporting clients in overseeing pressure, uneasiness, and keeping up with in general mental prosperity. These applications frequently incorporate highlights, for example, directed contemplation, care works out, mind-set following, and unwinding methods. Some emotional wellness applications likewise give assets to rest improvement, stress decrease, and survival techniques for different psychological well-being conditions.

**Rest Following and Improvement:**

Rest following applications intend to screen and dissect clients' rest examples to give experiences into the quality and length of their rest. These applications might utilize sensors in cell phones or wearables to distinguish development, survey rest stages, and give proposals for further developing rest cleanliness. Clients can get to information on their rest cycles, put forth rest objectives, and get ideas for upgrading their rest schedules.

**Ladies' Wellbeing Following:**

Ladies' wellbeing applications take care of explicit requirements connected with feminine cycle following, richness, and pregnancy. These applications frequently incorporate elements for logging feminine cycles, anticipating ovulation, and checking richness windows. With regards to pregnancy, some applications give direction on pre-birth care, child improvement, and post pregnancy health.

**Ongoing Infection The executives:**

Wellbeing and health applications assume a critical part in the administration of persistent illnesses like diabetes, hypertension, and cardiovascular circumstances. These applications empower clients to screen indispensable signs, track medicine adherence, and get customized care plans. By working with remote observing, these applications add to proactive sickness the executives and early mediation, further developing in general wellbeing results.

**Telehealth Administrations:**

Telehealth applications carry medical care administrations to clients' fingertips by offering virtual conferences with medical services experts. These applications frequently incorporate video conferencing highlights, secure informing, and the capacity to remotely impart wellbeing data to medical services suppliers. Telehealth administrations improve admittance to clinical guidance, work with follow-up counsels, and diminish obstructions to medical services, especially in circumstances where in-person visits might challenge.

**Advantages of Wellbeing and Health Applications:**

The advantages of wellbeing and health applications are different and add to encouraging a proactive and drew in way to deal with individual prosperity. A portion of the key benefits include:

**Accommodation and Openness:**

Wellbeing and wellbeing applications furnish clients with helpful admittance to an abundance of wellbeing related data and assets. Clients can screen their wellbeing, access customized bits of knowledge, and get direction without the requirements of time or area. This comfort advances ordinary commitment with wellbeing related exercises, adding to a more proactive way to deal with prosperity.

**Personalization and Custom-made Mediations:**

Numerous wellbeing and wellbeing applications influence information examination and man-made reasoning to customize intercessions in view of individual wellbeing profiles. This personalization improves the pertinence and viability of wellbeing proposals, making them more custom-made to clients' particular necessities, inclinations, and wellbeing objectives.

**Strengthening and Self-Administration:**

Wellbeing and wellbeing applications enable people to partake in the administration of their wellbeing effectively. Clients can keep tabs on their development, put forth objectives, and arrive at informed conclusions about their way of life, work-out schedules, and dietary decisions. This feeling of strengthening cultivates a proactive mentality towards wellbeing, empowering clients to take responsibility for prosperity.

**Preventive Consideration and Early Intercession:**

The ceaseless observing capacities of wellbeing and health applications add to preventive consideration by empowering early location of deviations from gauge wellbeing measurements. Clients can get ideal alarms or bits of knowledge that speedy them to look for clinical consideration or make acclimations to their wellbeing schedules. This preventive methodology diminishes the gamble of inconveniences and adds to better long haul wellbeing results.

**Support for Persistent Sickness The executives:**

Wellbeing and health applications assume a urgent part in supporting people with persistent sicknesses in dealing with their circumstances. These applications work with remote checking, drug adherence, and correspondence with medical care suppliers. By giving devices to self-administration, these applications enable people to participate in the everyday administration of constant circumstances, prompting worked on personal satisfaction effectively.

**Local area Commitment and Social Help:**

Some wellbeing and wellbeing applications consolidate local area includes that permit clients to associate with other people who share comparable wellbeing objectives or conditions. These virtual networks give a stage to sharing encounters, looking for guidance, and encouraging social help. The feeling of local area commitment can improve inspiration, urge adherence to wellbeing schedules, and establish a strong climate for people pursuing normal wellbeing targets.

**Difficulties and Contemplations:**

While wellbeing and health applications offer huge advantages, they additionally face difficulties and contemplations that need cautious consideration for capable and viable execution:

**Information Security and Protection:**

The assortment and capacity of wellbeing related information in applications raise critical worries about information security and protection. Clients endow delicate data, including wellbeing measurements and individual subtleties, to these applications. Guaranteeing hearty safety efforts, consistence with protection guidelines, and straightforward correspondence about information taking care of practices are basic to fabricate and keep up with client trust.

**Quality and Dependability:**

The quality and dependability of wellbeing and health applications can fluctuate generally. Some applications might need logical approval, and their proposals may not be proof based. Guaranteeing that applications stick to laid out principles, giving exact data, and trying not to misdirect claims are vital contemplations for clients and medical services experts depending on these instruments.

**Interoperability and Joining:**

Interoperability stays a test in the wellbeing application environment. Numerous applications work autonomously, prompting divided wellbeing records and deficient client profiles. Accomplishing consistent mix between various applications and stages, as well as similarity with electronic wellbeing records (EHRs), is fundamental for making a brought together and complete perspective on clients' wellbeing.

**Client Commitment and Adherence:**

Supporting client commitment and elevating long haul adherence to wellbeing and health applications can challenge. Client weakness, loss of interest, or absent mindedness might influence reliable application use. Planning applications with easy to use interfaces, consolidating gamification components, and offering continuous help and support are techniques to improve client commitment and adherence.

**Computerized Separation and Openness:**

The advanced separation presents difficulties connected with the openness of wellbeing and health applications. Not all people have equivalent admittance to cell phones, wearables, or dependable web availability. Addressing these variations is fundamental to forestall the intensification of existing medical services imbalances. Drives to give reasonable gadgets, advance computerized education, and plan comprehensive applications are basic for guaranteeing wide openness.

**Administrative Consistence:**

The administrative scene for wellbeing and health applications is advancing, and adherence to provincial and worldwide guidelines is fundamental. Engineers and suppliers should explore complex administrative structures, including information security regulations and clinical gadget guidelines. Remaining informed about administrative updates and effectively captivating in consistence measures are essential for mindful application advancement and sending.

**Influence on Medical services Environment:**

The inescapable reception of wellbeing and wellbeing applications prominently affects the more extensive medical care biological system. A few critical parts of this effect include:

**Shift Towards Patient-Driven Care:**

Wellbeing and health applications add to a change in perspective towards patient-driven care. By enabling people to effectively partake in the administration of their wellbeing, these applications line up with the standards of patient commitment and shared direction. Clients become accomplices in their medical services venture, cultivating a more cooperative relationship with medical care suppliers.

**Improved Admittance to Preventive Consideration:**

The constant checking and early mediation abilities of wellbeing and health applications upgrade admittance to preventive consideration. Clients can get opportune cautions or experiences that instant them to look for clinical consideration or make way of life changes. This proactive methodology adds to the anticipation of illnesses and entanglements, prompting further developed by and large wellbeing results.

**Support for Distant Patient Checking:**

Wellbeing and health applications assume a critical part in supporting far off understanding observing, especially with regards to constant sickness the board. These applications empower medical services suppliers to screen patients' wellbeing measurements from a distance, working with proactive mediations and decreasing the requirement for successive in-person visits. This help for remote observing adds to more proficient medical care conveyance.

**Joining with Telehealth Administrations:**

Numerous wellbeing and wellbeing applications coordinate with telehealth administrations, further extending admittance to medical services. Clients can flawlessly change from observing their wellbeing measurements on an application to taking part in virtual discussions with medical services experts. This reconciliation upgrades the continuum of care, giving a strong and associated medical services insight for clients.

**Information Driven Medical services Choices:**

The information produced by wellbeing and wellbeing applications add to information driven medical services choices. Medical services suppliers can use this data to acquire bits of knowledge into clients' wellbeing situations with, patterns, and designer intercessions in light of continuous information. This information driven approach improves the accuracy and personalization of medical care conveyance.

**4.2 Analysis of features such as symptom tracking, medication reminders, and mental health**

**support**

The combination of elements, for example, side effect following, drug updates, and emotional wellness support inside wellbeing and health applications addresses a urgent progression in utilizing innovation for all encompassing prosperity.

These highlights add to a more complete and customized way to deal with medical care, engaging clients to effectively deal with their wellbeing, stick to therapy plans, and address mental prosperity. This examination investigates the importance, advantages, challenges, and moral contemplations related with these vital highlights in wellbeing and health applications.

**Side effect Following:**

Side effect following elements in wellbeing and health applications furnish clients with a device to screen and keep changes in their physical or emotional well-being methodiclly. This usefulness is especially significant for people overseeing ongoing circumstances, going through treatment, or looking for bits of knowledge into designs that might influence their general prosperity.

**Benefits:**

**Early Discovery and Mediation:** Side effect following empowers early location of changes or patterns in medical issue. Clients can log side effects, track their recurrence and seriousness, and offer this data with medical care suppliers. Early recognition takes into consideration ideal mediations, possibly forestalling the heightening of medical problems.

**Objective Information for Medical care Suppliers:** By keeping an exhaustive record of side effects, clients furnish medical care suppliers with significant, objective information. This information supports more educated clinical direction, works with exact findings, and adds to customized treatment plans.

**Client Strengthening:** Side effect following enables clients by encouraging a more profound comprehension of their wellbeing. Perceiving examples and connections among's side effects and different variables, like way of life decisions or natural impacts, empowers clients to come to informed conclusions about their wellbeing and draw in proactively in their consideration.

**Challenges:**

**Information Exactness and Consistency:** The precision and consistency of side effect following rely upon clients' constancy and accuracy in logging data. Incorrect or fragmented information might upset the viability of side effect examination, influencing the nature of bits of knowledge acquired by medical services suppliers.

**Client Exhaustion and Consistence:** Steady and long haul side effect following requires client responsibility. In any case, clients might encounter exhaustion or separation after some time, influencing the unwavering quality of the information. Planning easy to understand interfaces, integrating updates, and utilizing gamification components can assist with alleviating these difficulties.

**Coordination with Other Wellbeing Information:** Side effect following is most important when incorporated with other wellbeing information, like indispensable signs or drug adherence. Interoperability difficulties might emerge while endeavoring to incorporate dissimilar wellsprings of wellbeing data, restricting the comprehensive perspective on client wellbeing.

**Medicine Updates:**

Drug update highlights in wellbeing and health applications act as a principal device for advancing medicine adherence, particularly for people overseeing ongoing circumstances or complex treatment regimens.

**Benefits:**

**Further developed Adherence:** Prescription updates essentially improve adherence to recommended treatment plans. Ordinary warnings and updates brief clients to accept drugs as endorsed, diminishing the gamble of missed portions and advancing the adequacy of restorative mediations.

**Customized Booking:** Clients can modify drug updates in light of their particular remedy plans. This personalization obliges varieties in medicine timing, measurement, and recurrence, lining up with individualized treatment plans.

**Combination with Wellbeing Records:** Numerous wellbeing and health applications incorporate prescription updates with electronic wellbeing records (EHRs) or other wellbeing following highlights. This reconciliation gives medical care suppliers continuous experiences into prescription adherence, supporting more exact evaluations and changes in accordance with therapy plans.

**Challenges:**

**Client Ready Exhaustion:** Persistent updates might prompt client weariness, where people become desensitized or irritated by successive warnings. Finding some kind of harmony between giving updates and keeping away from ready weariness requires smart plan and client criticism systems.

**Complex Therapy Regimens:** A few clients might have complex medicine regimens including numerous prescriptions with various timetables. Planning update frameworks that oblige these intricacies while residual easy to use is a test.

**Protection and Security:** Drug data is touchy, and clients might have worries about the security and security of their medicine information. Guaranteeing vigorous information safety efforts and straightforward correspondence about protection rehearses are fundamental for building client trust.

**Psychological well-being Backing:**

The joining of emotional wellness support highlights in wellbeing and health applications recognizes the interconnected idea of physical and mental prosperity. These elements include a scope of devices and assets pointed toward advancing mental wellbeing, stress the board, and in general profound wellbeing.

**Benefits:**

**Available Psychological well-being Assets:** Emotional wellness support highlights give clients effectively open assets for overseeing pressure, nervousness, and other psychological well-being concerns. Directed reflection, care activities, and unwinding procedures add to a comprehensive way to deal with prosperity.

**Disgrace Decrease:** By consolidating emotional well-being support inside standard wellbeing and health applications, there is potential to diminish the shame related with looking for psychological well-being help. Clients might feel more open to getting to these assets inside the recognizable setting of a more extensive wellbeing application.

**Thorough Prosperity:** Tending to psychological well-being in wellbeing and health applications perceives the significance of comprehensive prosperity. Clients can profit from a more thorough comprehension of the variables impacting their well-being, enveloping both physical and mental perspectives.

**Challenges:**

**Personalization and Various Requirements:** Emotional well-being is a profoundly private and different part of prosperity. Planning highlights that take care of a great many individual necessities and inclinations, while guaranteeing personalization, represents a test. Fitting emotional well-being backing to different client profiles requires a nuanced approach.

**Joining with Clinical Help:** While applications can offer significant assets for emotional well-being support, they are not a substitute for proficient clinical consideration. Incorporating these elements with components for associating clients to proficient emotional wellness administrations is significant to guarantee exhaustive help.

**Information Responsiveness and Moral Contemplations:** Psychological well-being information is especially touchy, and clients might have uplifted worries about protection. Guaranteeing moral information taking care of works on, getting educated assent, and straightforwardly conveying about information use are essential contemplations.

**Moral Contemplations:**

The joining of highlights, for example, side effect following, medicine updates, and psychological well-being support in wellbeing and health applications presents moral contemplations that request cautious consideration.

**Informed Assent and Client Independence:** Clients should give informed agree to the assortment and utilization of delicate wellbeing data, including side effects and psychological well-being information. Regarding client independence includes straightforwardly imparting how information will be utilized and giving clients the capacity to control and repudiate admittance to their data.

**Information Security and Protection:** Given the delicate idea of wellbeing information, guaranteeing vigorous information safety efforts is vital. Wellbeing and health applications should comply with security guidelines, for example, the Medical coverage Versatility and Responsibility Act (HIPAA) or the Overall Information Insurance Guideline (GDPR), to defend client protection and keep up with trust.

**Keeping away from Slander:** While tending to emotional well-being, application designers should endeavor to make includes that destigmatize looking for help for mental prosperity. Language, symbolism, and generally speaking informing ought to add to a positive and comprehensive climate, empowering clients to use emotional wellness assets unafraid of judgment.

**Guaranteeing Precision and Proof Based Practices:** Side effect following and emotional wellness support highlights ought to be founded on exact data and proof based rehearses. Designers should guarantee that proposals and mediations line up with laid out clinical rules to stay away from deception and likely damage.

**Client Strengthening in Navigation:** Clients ought to have command over how their wellbeing information is utilized and shared. Giving clear choices to selecting in or quitting explicit highlights, as well as teaching clients about the ramifications of their decisions, enables them in the dynamic cycle with respect to their wellbeing data.

**4.3 Discussion on the role of data privacy and security in health apps**

The job of information protection and security in wellbeing applications is vital, given the delicate idea of individual wellbeing data. As innovation keeps on propelling, wellbeing applications have become fundamental apparatuses in the medical care scene, offering clients elements, for example, side effect following, prescription updates, and emotional well-being support. Nonetheless, with the advantages come critical obligations to protect client information, guaranteeing security and security at each phase of information taking care of. This conversation dives into the basic parts of information protection and security in wellbeing applications, analyzing their significance, challenges, and moral contemplations.

**Significance of Information Protection and Security:**

**Defending Delicate Wellbeing Data:**

Wellbeing applications manage delicate and individual wellbeing data, including side effects, meds, and emotional well-being information. Safeguarding this data is pivotal for legitimate and administrative consistence as well as for keeping up with client trust. Clients depend wellbeing applications with their most confidential information, and any split the difference in protection could have serious results.

**Consistence with Guidelines:**

Adherence to information security guidelines is required for wellbeing applications. Contingent upon the area, guidelines, for example, the Medical coverage Movability and Responsibility Act (HIPAA) in the US or the Overall Information Security Guideline (GDPR) in Europe set severe principles for the assurance of wellbeing related information. Rebelliousness can prompt legitimate outcomes and harm the standing of wellbeing application designers.

**Client Trust and Reception:**

Client trust is primary for the achievement and boundless reception of wellbeing applications. At the point when clients genuinely trust the protection and safety efforts carried out by an application, they are bound to connect reliably and share exact data. Trust is particularly vital in the medical care area, where the results of information breaks can be extreme.

**Forestalling Unapproved Access:**

Unapproved admittance to wellbeing information presents huge dangers.

Information breaks can prompt wholesale fraud, extortion, or even the split the difference of individual wellbeing records. Carrying out strong safety efforts, including encryption and access controls, is fundamental to keep unapproved parties from getting to delicate wellbeing data.

### Challenges in Information Protection and Security:
### Interoperability Issues:

Interoperability challenges emerge when wellbeing applications need to trade information with other applications or medical services frameworks. Guaranteeing that information is safely sent and gotten across various stages without compromising protection can challenge. Normalization endeavors are progressing to resolve this issue.

### Client Confirmation and Approval:

Laying out secure client verification cycles and approval instruments is basic. Feeble passwords or insufficient access controls can prompt unapproved access. Executing multifaceted validation and strong client approval conventions mitigates these dangers.

### Information Encryption and Unscrambling:

Scrambling wellbeing information during transmission and capacity is a principal security measure. In any case, the most common way of encoding and decoding information should be all around carried out to keep away from weaknesses. Guaranteeing that encryption keys are secure and dealing with the encryption/decoding process actually are progressing difficulties.

### Outsider Coordination Dangers:

Numerous wellbeing applications coordinate with outsider administrations or gadgets, for example, wearables or electronic wellbeing record frameworks. Guaranteeing that these combinations are secure and agreeable with protection guidelines presents difficulties. Application designers should completely vet and screen outsider accomplices to limit expected chances.

### Information Capacity Practices:

How wellbeing information is put away, whether on neighborhood gadgets or in the cloud, has suggestions for protection and security. Secure capacity rehearses include measures, for example, information anonymization, customary security reviews, and adherence to industry best practices in information maintenance and removal.

### Moral Contemplations:
### Informed Assent:

Acquiring informed assent is a moral basic in wellbeing applications. Clients should be plainly educated about how their wellbeing information will be utilized, shared, and put away. Straightforwardness in information rehearses guarantees that clients are arriving at informed conclusions about the degree to which they will share their delicate wellbeing data.

### Client Control and Independence:

Regarding client independence includes giving clients command over their information. Wellbeing applications ought to offer clients choices to deal with their protection settings, including the capacity to pick in or quit explicit highlights. Clients ought to be engaged to come to conclusions about the utilization of their wellbeing information in a manner that lines up with their inclinations.

**Keeping away from Shady Practices:**

Moral wellbeing applications focus on the prosperity of clients over manipulative practices. Information ought to be utilized to help clients instead of for purposes that might take advantage of weaknesses or lead to hurt. Designers should comply with moral rules, staying away from rehearses that could think twice about security or control wellbeing data for ulterior intentions.

**Clear Correspondence:**

Moral wellbeing applications keep up with clear and straightforward correspondence with clients. This includes giving available and reasonable protection arrangements, terms of purpose, and clarifications of information rehearses. Guaranteeing that clients are very much informed cultivates trust and advances a positive connection among clients and the wellbeing application.

**Best Practices for Information Protection and Security:**

**Start to finish Encryption:**

Executing start to finish encryption guarantees that information is safely communicated from the client's gadget to the server as well as the other way around. This forestalls unapproved admittance to information during transmission and safeguards delicate wellbeing data from interference.

**Standard Security Reviews:**

Directing standard security reviews is fundamental to recognize and address expected weaknesses. These reviews ought to envelop both the application's codebase and its framework. Standard testing guarantees that the application stays tough against advancing security dangers.

**Information Minimization:**

Sticking to the rule of information minimization includes gathering just the important data expected for the application's usefulness. Pointless information assortment expands the gamble related with information breaks and security infringement. Restricting information assortment to what is fundamental improves both protection and security.

**Client Schooling:**

Instructing clients about the significance of information protection and security advances dependable utilization. Giving clear data on how their information will be dealt with, the safety efforts set up, and steps they can take to improve their own security mindfulness adds to a more educated client base.

**Consistence with Guidelines:**

Keeping up to date with and consenting to significant information security guidelines is a central best practice. This incorporates understanding the lawful necessities pertinent to wellbeing applications in unambiguous areas and guaranteeing that the application's arrangements line up with these guidelines.

**4.4 Showcasing innovative health platforms connecting users and healthcare professionals**

As of late, the medical care scene has seen an extraordinary shift with the rise of creative wellbeing stages that encourage consistent associations among clients and medical care experts. These stages influence trend setting innovations to upgrade availability, work with correspondence, and engage people to effectively participate in their medical services venture. This conversation investigates a few striking instances of these inventive wellbeing stages, featuring their elements, benefits, and the ground-breaking effect they bring to the medical services biological system.

**Telehealth Stages:**

Telehealth stages have arisen as a foundation of present day medical care, offering virtual interviews and far off medical services administrations. These stages empower clients to associate with medical care experts from the solace of their homes, wiping out geological hindrances and improving admittance to clinical skill. With highlights, for example, video conferencing, secure informing, and electronic wellbeing record mix, telehealth stages work with ongoing correspondence and empower medical services suppliers to remotely analyze, screen, and treat a great many ailments.

One of the critical advantages of telehealth stages is the comfort they give to clients. People can look for clinical guidance without the requirement for in-person visits, lessening travel time and related costs. Also, telehealth stages have demonstrated priceless in circumstances where actual admittance to medical services offices might be restricted, as seen during worldwide wellbeing emergencies.

**Wellbeing Data Trade Stages:**

Wellbeing data trade (HIE) stages assume a critical part in working on the interoperability and sharing of wellbeing information among various medical care substances. These stages empower secure and normalized trade of patient data, encouraging joint effort between medical services experts across different settings. By giving a brought together perspective on persistent wellbeing records, HIE stages improve care coordination, diminish duplication of tests and strategies, and eventually add to better quiet results.

The advantages of HIE stages stretch out past individual experiences with medical care experts. They support thorough and longitudinal patient consideration by guaranteeing that applicable wellbeing data is accessible to approved experts at the mark of care. This consistent trade of data upgrades the precision of judgments, further develops medicine the executives, and elevates a comprehensive way to deal with medical services conveyance.

**Distant Patient Checking Stages:**

Far off understanding observing (RPM) stages influence associated gadgets to follow and send continuous wellbeing information from patients to medical services suppliers. These stages are especially effective for people overseeing persistent circumstances or recuperating from medical procedures. Through wearable gadgets and sensors, RPM stages constantly screen fundamental signs, movement levels, and other important wellbeing measurements, permitting medical services experts to remotely evaluate patients' prosperity.

RPM stages add to proactive medical services by empowering early discovery of changes in wellbeing status. For instance, with regards to persistent illnesses like diabetes or hypertension, RPM stages engage medical care suppliers to mediate speedily because of deviations from typical wellbeing boundaries. This proactive methodology decreases the gamble of difficulties, limits emergency clinic readmissions, and upgrades by and large tolerant consideration.

**Patient Commitment Stages:**

Patient commitment stages center around engaging people to effectively take part in their medical care venture. These stages offer highlights, for example, customized wellbeing data, arrangement booking, drug updates, and intelligent instructive assets. By cultivating correspondence among patients and medical services suppliers, patient commitment stages plan to upgrade wellbeing proficiency, further develop therapy adherence, and fortify the patient-supplier relationship.

The intuitive idea of patient commitment stages urges clients to play a more proactive job in dealing with their wellbeing. Patients can get to significant data, track their wellbeing measurements, and speak with their medical care group through secure informing highlights. This expanded commitment adds to better-educated direction, further developed treatment results, and a feeling of strengthening among clients.

**Difficulties and Contemplations:**

While these creative wellbeing stages offer critical benefits, they likewise face difficulties that require cautious thought. Protection and security concerns, interoperability issues, and the requirement for administrative consistence are normal difficulties across these stages. Guaranteeing that client information is safeguarded, cultivating interoperability between various frameworks, and exploring complex administrative scenes are continuous needs for engineers and medical services suppliers.

Besides, the computerized partition stays a test, with variations in admittance to innovation and web network influencing specific populaces. Endeavors to address these differences, for example, giving reasonable gadgets and advancing computerized proficiency, are fundamental to guarantee that the advantages of these stages are open to a different scope of clients.

# Chapter 5

## Artificial Intelligence in Health Monitoring

Computerized reasoning (man-made intelligence) has arisen as a groundbreaking power across different ventures, and its effect on medical services is especially significant. As of late, there has been a developing accentuation on utilizing computer based intelligence for wellbeing observing, changing the manner in which we track and deal with our prosperity. This coordination of cutting edge innovation into medical services frameworks holds the possibility to improve diagnostics, customized therapy plans, and by and large understanding results.

One of the key regions where simulated intelligence is taking huge steps is in wellbeing checking gadgets. Wearable innovation, for example, smartwatches and wellness trackers, outfitted with artificial intelligence calculations, has become progressively famous. These gadgets go past conventional wellness following, developing into exhaustive wellbeing screens able to do consistently gathering and examining different physiological boundaries.

Simulated intelligence controlled wellbeing checking gadgets can follow measurements like pulse, rest designs, and actual work with exceptional precision. The ongoing information produced by these gadgets furnish people and medical services experts with significant bits of knowledge into a singular's general wellbeing. For instance, anomalies in pulse examples or disturbances in rest cycles might show potential medical problems, provoking ideal mediation.

Additionally, computer based intelligence adds to the personalization of wellbeing checking. The capacity of artificial intelligence calculations to learn and adjust to a singular's interesting physiology takes into consideration more customized and exact wellbeing evaluations. This degree of customization is essential, as it recognizes the intrinsic variety in human science and guarantees that wellbeing proposals are custom-made to the particular necessities of every person.

Notwithstanding wearables, artificial intelligence is likewise being coordinated into conventional clinical gadgets to upgrade wellbeing observing abilities. For example, simulated intelligence calculations can dissect clinical imaging information, like X-beams and X-rays, to identify unpretentious anomalies that might be characteristic of beginning phase illnesses. This early recognition works on the possibilities of effective treatment as well as diminishes the weight on medical care frameworks by forestalling the movement of illnesses to cutting edge stages.

The utilization of artificial intelligence in wellbeing checking reaches out past individual gadgets. Coordinated medical care environments are arising, where information from different sources, including wearables, electronic wellbeing records, and indicative tests, are accumulated and examined all things considered. This all encompassing way to deal with wellbeing observing gives an exhaustive perspective on a singular's wellbeing, empowering a more proactive and preventive medical services model.

In any case, the boundless reception of artificial intelligence in wellbeing checking accompanies its own arrangement of difficulties. Protection and security concerns are at the very front, as the assortment and examination of individual wellbeing information bring up moral issues. Finding some kind of harmony between using computer based intelligence for further developed wellbeing results and defending individual security is a basic thought that requires cautious administrative structures and mechanical shields.

Another test is the requirement for interoperability among various wellbeing checking gadgets and frameworks. As the medical services scene turns out to be progressively digitized, guaranteeing that different simulated intelligence fueled gadgets can consistently impart and share information is fundamental. Normalized conventions and open-source structures assume a critical part in defeating interoperability challenges, cultivating a more associated and proficient medical services biological system.

The combination of simulated intelligence in wellbeing checking likewise brings up issues about the job of medical care experts. While artificial intelligence can examine huge measures of information and produce significant experiences, the human touch stays indispensable in understanding consideration. Medical care suppliers should adjust to a cooperative model where man-made intelligence expands their capacities as opposed to supplanting them. This requires continuous schooling and preparing to guarantee that medical services experts are capable in utilizing artificial intelligence devices to improve patient consideration.

The expected advantages of artificial intelligence in wellbeing checking reach out past individual patient consideration to populace wellbeing the executives. By breaking down collected information from enormous populaces, computer based intelligence can recognize patterns, risk variables, and likely flare-ups. This populace level examination empowers medical care frameworks to carry out designated intercessions and preventive measures, eventually working on the general wellbeing of networks.

In the domain of constant sickness the board, computer based intelligence assumes a crucial part in giving nonstop checking and customized mediations. For people with constant circumstances, for example, diabetes or hypertension, simulated intelligence controlled frameworks can break down ongoing information to distinguish examples and patterns. This data can be utilized to change treatment plans, suggest way of life adjustments, and anticipate intensifications, prompting better sickness the executives and worked on personal satisfaction.

The utilization of artificial intelligence in wellbeing observing isn't restricted to actual wellbeing; it additionally stretches out to psychological well-being. Psychological wellness problems are a huge worldwide wellbeing trouble, and early discovery is frequently difficult. Computer based intelligence calculations can break down designs in discourse, conduct, and, surprisingly, online entertainment action to identify expected indications of psychological wellness issues. This proactive way to deal with psychological well-being observing considers convenient mediations, decreasing the disgrace related with emotional wellness and working on generally speaking prosperity.

Moreover, man-made intelligence adds to the democratization of medical care by growing admittance to observing and analytic administrations. Telehealth stages, controlled by simulated intelligence, empower people to get far off counsels and checking, separating geological hindrances and expanding admittance to medical care administrations, especially in underserved or distant regions.

As artificial intelligence keeps on developing, the coordination of cutting edge innovations, for example, regular language handling and prescient examination further improves its capacities in wellbeing observing. Regular language handling empowers man-made intelligence frameworks to comprehend and decipher human language, working with additional normal and instinctive collaborations. This is especially significant in virtual wellbeing colleagues and chatbots that can draw in with people to assemble wellbeing data and give important experiences.

Prescient investigation, then again, use authentic information and AI calculations to conjecture future wellbeing results. With regards to wellbeing checking, prescient examination can distinguish people at higher gamble of creating explicit circumstances, taking into account designated preventive measures. This proactive methodology lines up with the shift from responsive medical services to an additional prescient and preventive model, at last decreasing the general medical care trouble.

As the coordination of man-made intelligence in wellbeing observing turns out to be more far and wide, the job of information administration becomes vital. The huge measures of information produced by wellbeing checking gadgets and frameworks require powerful administration structures to guarantee dependable and moral use.

Clear rules on information proprietorship, assent, and straightforwardness are crucial for construct trust among people and encourage a cooperative biological system between innovation engineers, medical care suppliers, and patients.

Furthermore, headways in man-made intelligence driven genomics are making ready for customized medication. Man-made intelligence calculations can examine genomic information to distinguish explicit hereditary markers related with infection risk, reaction to treatment, and likely aftereffects. This degree of genomic investigation considers the advancement of designated treatments, limiting unfriendly impacts and improving treatment results.

The joining of computer based intelligence in genomics additionally adds to progressions in accuracy medication. By consolidating genomic information with other wellbeing related data, artificial intelligence can recognize examples and connections that guide the choice of the best medicines for individual patients. This shift towards accuracy medication addresses a paradigmatic change in medical services, creating some distance from one-size-fits-all ways to deal with profoundly customized and designated mediations.

With regards to irresistible illnesses, man-made intelligence has demonstrated to be an important device in checking and controlling flare-ups. During worldwide wellbeing emergencies, for example, the Coronavirus pandemic, computer based intelligence calculations have been utilized to examine epidemiological information, track the spread of the infection, and anticipate expected areas of interest. This constant examination empowers general wellbeing specialists to carry out designated intercessions, allot assets productively, and moderate the effect of the episode.

Nonetheless, the mix of computer based intelligence in wellbeing observing isn't without challenges and moral contemplations. The potential for predisposition in computer based intelligence calculations, especially in genomic examination, is a worry that should be tended to. One-sided calculations might prompt abberations in medical services results, building up existing disparities. Thorough testing, approval, and continuous checking of man-made intelligence calculations are fundamental to guarantee that they are fair, unprejudiced, and agent of different populaces.

The moral utilization of computer based intelligence in wellbeing observing likewise reaches out to issues of assent and information proprietorship. People should have command over their wellbeing information, with clear instruments for giving informed assent and quitting information sharing. Straightforward correspondence with respect to how wellbeing information will be utilized and shared is vital to building trust between people, medical care suppliers, and innovation designers.

The fate of artificial intelligence in wellbeing checking holds the commitment of nonstop development and improvement. The improvement of further developed sensors, combined with progressively modern man-made intelligence calculations, will additionally upgrade the exactness and granularity of wellbeing information gathered. This, thus, will empower more exact diagnostics, early location of medical problems, and customized therapy plans.

Besides, the reconciliation of computer based intelligence with arising innovations like the Web of Things (IoT) will make a more interconnected and smart medical services environment. IoT gadgets, going from savvy home machines to clinical inserts, can speak with man-made intelligence frameworks to give a comprehensive perspective on a singular's wellbeing. For instance, a shrewd fridge could follow dietary propensities, and an associated pacemaker could communicate continuous heart information, all adding to a thorough wellbeing profile.

The intermingling of man-made intelligence, IoT, and 5G innovation will additionally speed up the advancement of ongoing wellbeing observing frameworks. The low-idleness capacities of 5G organizations empower consistent correspondence between gadgets, guaranteeing that wellbeing information is sent and broke down in close to constant. This immediate criticism circle is especially essential in crisis circumstances or for people with intense ailments, considering quick mediations and further developed results.

As artificial intelligence in wellbeing observing advances, the job of administrative bodies turns out to be progressively significant. Administrative structures should develop to stay up with innovative progressions, guaranteeing that man-made intelligence controlled wellbeing checking gadgets and frameworks fulfill severe guidelines for security, adequacy, and information protection. Cooperation between administrative specialists, industry partners, and the clinical local area is fundamental to lay out rules that cultivate advancement while shielding patient interests.

The mix of computer based intelligence in wellbeing checking additionally carries financial contemplations into the spotlight. While the underlying interest in artificial intelligence advances might be significant, the drawn out benefits as far as further developed wellbeing results, decreased medical care costs, and expanded effectiveness are critical. Legislatures, medical services suppliers, and guarantors should team up to foster maintainable models that boost the reception of artificial intelligence in wellbeing checking and guarantee evenhanded admittance to these advancements.

### 5.1 Exploration of AI applications in analyzing health data

The field of man-made consciousness (computer based intelligence) has seen astounding progressions, and its applications in medical care, especially in the examination of wellbeing information, are turning out to be progressively pervasive. The investigation of artificial intelligence in medical care information examination holds the commitment of changing how clinical data is deciphered, prompting more exact determinations, customized therapy designs, and worked on understanding results.

Wellbeing information, in its different structures, is an immense and complex asset that incorporates electronic wellbeing records (EHRs), clinical imaging, genomic information, and constant physiological checking. The sheer volume and variety of wellbeing information present the two difficulties and amazing open doors for medical care experts. This is where man-made intelligence arises as a strong partner, equipped for handling, examining, and extricating significant experiences from monstrous datasets in manners that were once unfathomable.

One conspicuous region where man-made intelligence succeeds in wellbeing information examination is clinical imaging. The translation of clinical pictures, for example, X-beams, CT sweeps, and X-rays, customarily depends on the mastery of radiologists. Nonetheless, the coordination of simulated intelligence calculations has altogether expanded the analytic capacities in this area. Man-made intelligence fueled picture examination can identify unpretentious irregularities, aid early illness discovery, and give quantitative evaluations exceptional precision.

For example, in the area of radiology, artificial intelligence calculations can quickly break down enormous arrangements of clinical pictures to distinguish designs characteristic of illnesses like malignant growth or neurological issues. The speed and effectiveness of man-made intelligence based picture investigation facilitate the indicative cycle as well as lessen the probability of human mistake. This cooperative methodology, where man-made intelligence goes about as a strong instrument for medical services experts, improves symptomatic accuracy and adds to more compelling patient consideration.

Past clinical imaging, man-made intelligence is taking significant steps in the examination of genomic information. Genomic medication, which includes the investigation of a person's hereditary data, can possibly upset medical care by empowering customized therapy plans in light of an individual's one of a kind hereditary cosmetics. Artificial intelligence calculations assume a pivotal part in unraveling the intricacies of genomic information, recognizing hereditary markers related with explicit illnesses, and foreseeing individual reactions to different medicines.

In disease exploration and treatment, computer based intelligence is being utilized to break down genomic information to recognize changes and modifications that drive cancer development. This data is instrumental in fitting designated treatments that are more powerful and less inclined to secondary effects than conventional medicines. The capacity of simulated intelligence to filter through immense genomic datasets continuously works with quick progressions in understanding the hereditary premise of illnesses, preparing for accuracy medication.

Ongoing physiological observing is another region where man-made intelligence applications are reshaping the scene of medical care. Wearable gadgets furnished with simulated intelligence calculations can persistently follow different wellbeing boundaries, for example, pulse, rest designs, and actual work. The information created by these gadgets give important bits of knowledge into a singular's general wellbeing and empower the early location of deviations from typical examples.

For instance, artificial intelligence controlled wearables can distinguish abnormalities in pulse designs that might demonstrate possible cardiovascular issues. Essentially, deviations in rest designs or abrupt changes in actual work levels could act as early advance notice finishes paperwork for different ailments. By giving constant checking and investigation, computer based intelligence empowered wearables engage people to go to proactive lengths for their prosperity and empower medical care experts to intercede at the earliest phases of potential medical problems.

In the domain of electronic wellbeing records (EHRs), man-made intelligence is smoothing out the examination of tremendous measures of patient information. EHRs contain far reaching data about a patient's clinical history, medicines, meds, and results. Computer based intelligence calculations can filter through this abundance of information to recognize examples, patterns, and relationships that may not be clear through conventional techniques.

One critical use of artificial intelligence in EHR examination is prescient investigation. By utilizing AI calculations, man-made intelligence can anticipate the probability of explicit wellbeing results in light of verifiable information. This proactive methodology empowers medical care suppliers to recognize high-risk patients, intercede early, and carry out preventive measures to work on understanding results and decrease medical services costs.

Computer based intelligence driven regular language handling (NLP) is likewise assuming a critical part in EHR examination. NLP calculations can separate significant data from unstructured clinical notes, empowering a more exhaustive comprehension of a patient's condition. This capacity upgrades the interoperability of wellbeing information and works with more powerful correspondence among medical services experts, at last prompting worked on understanding consideration.

The reconciliation of computer based intelligence in wellbeing information examination reaches out to the field of medication disclosure and advancement. The customary medication improvement process is tedious and expensive, with a high pace of disappointment. Computer based intelligence offers a groundbreaking methodology by speeding up the ID of potential medication competitors, foreseeing their viability, and enhancing treatment regimens.

Artificial intelligence calculations can dissect tremendous datasets, including natural and synthetic data, to distinguish potential medication targets and foresee the organic action of new mixtures. This information driven approach speeds up the beginning phases of medication revelation, lessening the time and assets expected to put up new medicines for sale to the public. In addition, computer based intelligence works with the distinguishing proof of patient subgroups that might answer distinctively to medicines, empowering the improvement of additional designated and customized treatments.

In clinical preliminaries, artificial intelligence is smoothing out the enlistment cycle by distinguishing qualified members in view of explicit standards. This speeds up the preliminary enlistment process as well as guarantees that different patient populaces are incorporated, prompting more vigorous and generalizable review results.

In spite of the massive capability of simulated intelligence in wellbeing information examination, a few difficulties should be addressed to boost its effect. Information protection and security are vital worries, particularly as wellbeing information turns out to be progressively digitized and interconnected. Severe guidelines and moral rules are crucial for defend patient data and guarantee mindful and straightforward utilization of man-made intelligence in medical services.

The issue of predisposition in computer based intelligence calculations is another basic thought. One-sided calculations might prompt abberations in medical care results, as they may not precisely address different patient populaces. Thorough testing, approval, and progressing checking are important to relieve predisposition and guarantee that simulated intelligence applications in wellbeing information examination are fair and impartial.

Interoperability among various medical services frameworks and information sources is another test that requires consideration. As man-made intelligence applications develop, consistent correspondence and information trade between different stages are fundamental to make an associated and cooperative medical services environment. Normalized conventions and open-source structures can add to conquering interoperability difficulties and encourage advancement.

The reconciliation of artificial intelligence in wellbeing information examination likewise requires a change in the jobs and obligations of medical care experts. It is essential to guarantee that medical care suppliers are furnished with the fundamental abilities to decipher and apply computer based intelligence produced experiences in clinical practice. This requires progressing instruction and preparing projects to overcome any barrier between customary clinical ability and the capacities of simulated intelligence advancements.

Also, viable correspondence between artificial intelligence frameworks and medical care experts is fundamental for the fruitful coordination of man-made intelligence in medical care work processes. Clear and interpretable clarifications of man-made intelligence created suggestions engage medical care suppliers to pursue informed choices and fabricate trust in the innovation. This human-man-made intelligence coordinated effort is critical to bridling the maximum capacity of artificial intelligence in wellbeing information examination.

Looking forward, the fate of artificial intelligence in wellbeing information examination holds energizing prospects. The continuous headways in AI, profound learning, and normal language handling will additionally upgrade the abilities of man-made intelligence calculations. This incorporates the advancement of more reasonable man-made intelligence models, empowering medical care experts to all the more likely comprehend and believe the proposals produced by these frameworks.

The union of computer based intelligence with other arising innovations, like the Web of Things (IoT) and 5G, will make a more interconnected and canny medical services biological system. IoT gadgets, going from wearable sensors to savvy clinical gadgets, can produce continuous information that artificial intelligence calculations break down for ideal experiences. The low-inertness capacities of 5G organizations guarantee quick and consistent correspondence between these gadgets and computer based intelligence frameworks, empowering a more responsive and productive medical services foundation.

**5.2 Discussion on the ethical considerations of using AI in health monitoring**

The reconciliation of man-made reasoning (artificial intelligence) in wellbeing checking achieves various advantages, from further developed diagnostics to customized treatment plans. In any case, this mechanical headway additionally raises moral contemplations that should be painstakingly addressed to guarantee dependable and evenhanded use. Looking at the moral components of artificial intelligence in wellbeing checking is fundamental as it includes the handling of delicate individual data, possible predispositions in calculations, and the changing elements of the patient-specialist relationship.

One of the essential moral worries in the utilization of artificial intelligence in wellbeing checking is the issue of protection. Wellbeing information, including data gathered through wearables, electronic wellbeing records, and other checking gadgets, is profoundly touchy and individual. The consistent, continuous nature of man-made intelligence empowered wellbeing observing implies that people are continually creating information about their physiological and standards of conduct. Finding some kind of harmony between using this information for medical services upgrades and safeguarding individual protection turns into a basic test.

To address these protection concerns, powerful administrative systems should be set up. Legitimate measures ought to command straightforward information rehearses, obviously framing how wellbeing information will be gathered, put away, and shared. People should be educated about the reason regarding information assortment, and express assent ought to be gotten. Furthermore, there ought to be systems set up for people to access, control, and even eradicate their wellbeing information assuming they decide to do as such.

Also, guaranteeing the security of wellbeing information is foremost. As man-made intelligence frameworks become more incorporated into medical care foundation, there is an expanded gamble of information breaks and digital assaults. Satisfactory network safety measures, including encryption and secure transmission conventions, are important to safeguard the privacy and respectability of wellbeing data. Foundations and associations taking care of wellbeing information should put resources into vigorous online protection framework to alleviate the dangers related with unapproved access.

One more moral thought in the utilization of man-made intelligence in wellbeing observing is the potential for predisposition in calculations. Man-made intelligence frameworks gain from authentic information, and assuming the preparation information is one-sided, the calculations can sustain and try and intensify existing inconsistencies. This is especially concerning with regards to wellbeing observing, as one-sided calculations might prompt erroneous forecasts or suggestions, affecting the nature of care conveyed to various segment gatherings.

To relieve predisposition in artificial intelligence calculations, it is pivotal to guarantee different and agent preparing datasets. Designers ought to be mindful of possible predispositions in information assortment and constantly evaluate and rethink algorithmic results to recognize and address any abberations. Furthermore, straightforwardness in the turn of events and arrangement of artificial intelligence frameworks is fundamental. Straightforwardly conveying about the calculations' limits, inclinations, and potential dangers encourages trust and considers outside investigation.

The straightforwardness of simulated intelligence frameworks reaches out past the specialized viewpoints to incorporate the logic of artificial intelligence produced proposals. Medical services experts and people being observed should have the option to comprehend how computer based intelligence calculations come to explicit end results or forecasts. The "discovery" nature of some computer based intelligence models can disintegrate trust, making it basic to foster interpretable man-made intelligence frameworks that give clear clarifications to their results.

Besides, the organization of simulated intelligence in wellbeing checking brings up issues about the job of medical care experts and the specialist patient relationship. While man-made intelligence can examine tremendous measures of information and create bits of knowledge, it misses the mark on sympathetic and human-driven approach that is vital to medical care. The moral utilization of computer based intelligence ought to stress a cooperative model where man-made intelligence improves the capacities of medical services experts instead of supplanting them.

Medical services suppliers should be satisfactorily prepared to decipher and apply artificial intelligence created experiences in clinical practice. The reconciliation of artificial intelligence into the work process ought to supplement the abilities and aptitude of medical services experts, permitting them to zero in on complex navigation, patient correspondence, and humane consideration. Keeping up with the human touch in medical services is critical to guarantee that people feel seen, heard, and grasped, encouraging a patient-focused approach.

The moral contemplations of man-made intelligence in wellbeing checking likewise reach out to the possible effect on weak populaces. Financial elements, admittance to innovation, and advanced proficiency can make differences in the capacity to profit from computer based intelligence empowered wellbeing checking. There is a gamble that specific gatherings might be abandoned, intensifying existing wellbeing disparities. Moral arrangement of computer based intelligence ought to focus on inclusivity, guaranteeing that the advantages of wellbeing checking advancements are available to assorted populaces.

In tending to these worries, policymakers and medical services associations ought to effectively pursue lessening the advanced gap. Drives that elevate fair admittance to innovation, give training on the best way to utilize simulated intelligence empowered wellbeing observing apparatuses, and guarantee reasonableness are fundamental. Furthermore, mediations ought to be planned with an emphasis on social capability, recognizing different points of view on wellbeing and prosperity.

The moral contemplations of simulated intelligence in wellbeing observing are entwined with more extensive cultural ramifications. As these advances become more imbued in medical services frameworks, questions emerge about their effect on work in the medical care area. The expanded effectiveness achieved by simulated intelligence might prompt changes in work jobs, possibly uprooting specific assignments customarily performed by people.

To address these worries, a capable and moral methodology includes expecting the effect of man-made intelligence on business and effectively pursuing upskilling and reskilling medical care experts. Preparing projects ought to be intended to outfit people with the abilities important to team up successfully with man-made intelligence frameworks, cultivating a labor force that can use innovation to improve patient consideration.

Moreover, a smart way to deal with man-made intelligence in wellbeing checking ought to think about the possible financial ramifications for people. The expense of man-made intelligence empowered wellbeing observing gadgets and administrations might make variations in access in light of financial status. Moral contemplations call for methodologies that guarantee reasonableness, possibly through endowments or protection inclusion, to forestall prohibition in light of monetary capacities.

With regards to psychological well-being checking, moral contemplations take on a particular aspect. Man-made intelligence calculations breaking down discourse designs, online entertainment movement, and other social markers for indications of emotional well-being issues raise worries about the delicate idea of emotional well-being information. Security and assent become considerably more basic, and people should have office over how their emotional wellness data is gathered, shared, and utilized.

Moreover, moral rules for psychological well-being observing utilizing man-made intelligence ought to focus on the prosperity of people. The distinguishing proof of potential psychological well-being issues ought to be joined by insightful mediations that focus on the person's emotional well-being and offer proper help. The joining of emotional well-being experts into the turn of events and sending of artificial intelligence in emotional wellness checking is fundamental to guarantee moral practices and stay away from expected hurt.

Looking forward, the moral contemplations of involving artificial intelligence in wellbeing observing will keep on developing close by mechanical headways. A proactive methodology includes continuous cooperation between policymakers, medical services experts, innovation designers, and ethicists. Persistent discourse, moral structures, and vigorous administrative measures are crucial for guide the mindful turn of events and arrangement of artificial intelligence in wellbeing checking, eventually guaranteeing that these advancements benefit people and society while maintaining basic moral standards.

### 5.3 Future trends and possibilities of AI-driven health technologies

The eventual fate of medical care is unpredictably attached to the proceeded with advancement of man-made reasoning (simulated intelligence)- driven innovations.

As we look forward, a few patterns and conceivable outcomes arise, promising to reshape the scene of medical care conveyance, diagnostics, and generally speaking patient results. From customized medication to expanded direction, the expected utilizations of artificial intelligence in medical services are immense and extraordinary.

One conspicuous future pattern in man-made intelligence driven wellbeing innovations is the headway of customized medication. The mix of man-made intelligence with genomics, proteomics, and other 'omics' information considers a more nuanced comprehension of individual wellbeing at the sub-atomic level. Artificial intelligence calculations can break down huge datasets, recognizing explicit hereditary markers and biomarkers related with illnesses and treatment reactions.

This degree of accuracy empowers medical care suppliers to fit therapy plans to individual patients, advancing remedial mediations in view of their exceptional hereditary cosmetics. The shift towards customized medication holds the commitment of expanded treatment adequacy, diminished aftereffects, and worked on persistent results. As man-made intelligence calculations become more capable at unraveling complex natural data, the time of really customized and designated medical services is not too far off.

One more future pattern is the far reaching reception of artificial intelligence in drug disclosure and improvement. Customary medication revelation processes are extensive and asset concentrated, with a high pace of disappointment. Simulated intelligence offers a progressive methodology by speeding up the ID of potential medication competitors, foreseeing their viability, and smoothing out the enhancement of treatment regimens.

Artificial intelligence calculations can break down huge datasets enveloping natural and synthetic data, working with the fast distinguishing proof of promising mixtures for additional review. This information driven approach not just facilitates the beginning phases of medication disclosure yet additionally empowers the advancement of additional designated treatments, lessening the time and assets expected to put up new medicines for sale to the public.

Notwithstanding drug revelation, man-made intelligence is ready to assume a critical part in clinical preliminary streamlining. Distinguishing qualified members, anticipating patient reactions, and improving preliminary conventions are regions where simulated intelligence can fundamentally affect the productivity and achievement paces of clinical preliminaries. By utilizing simulated intelligence to investigate different datasets, including patient socioeconomics, hereditary data, and certifiable proof, specialists can plan more comprehensive and successful preliminaries.

Distant patient observing, controlled by simulated intelligence, is another future pattern that holds incredible potential. The joining of wearable gadgets, sensors, and persistent checking advancements takes into consideration constant information assortment on different physiological boundaries. Man-made intelligence calculations can investigate this information, giving experiences into patterns, distinguishing irregularities, and working with early intercession.

For constant illness the executives, remote observing offers a proactive methodology. People with conditions like diabetes, hypertension, or coronary illness can profit from nonstop simulated intelligence driven observing that distinguishes unobtrusive changes in wellbeing measurements. This empowers medical care suppliers to make ideal acclimations to therapy plans, decreasing the gamble of inconveniences and further developing generally sickness the board.

The eventual fate of artificial intelligence driven wellbeing innovations additionally remembers headways for normal language handling (NLP) and conversational man-made intelligence. Virtual wellbeing collaborators and chatbots outfitted with modern NLP calculations can draw in with people to accumulate wellbeing data, give instructive assets, and, surprisingly, offer help for emotional well-being concerns.

Conversational artificial intelligence can possibly upgrade patient commitment and further develop wellbeing proficiency. People can collaborate with computer based intelligence fueled frameworks in a more regular and natural way, getting clarification on pressing issues, looking for direction, and getting customized wellbeing data. This not just engages people to play a functioning job in their wellbeing yet in addition works with more compelling correspondence among patients and medical services suppliers.

The union of simulated intelligence with the Web of Things (IoT) and 5G innovation is a future pattern that will additionally reform medical care. IoT gadgets, going from shrewd clinical gadgets to locally established sensors, can gather constant wellbeing information. The low-inertness capacities of 5G organizations empower consistent correspondence between these gadgets and man-made intelligence frameworks, considering fast investigation and reaction.

This interconnected medical services biological system holds the commitment of more productive and responsive medical care conveyance. Wearable gadgets can send information to simulated intelligence calculations that investigate patterns, distinguish anomalies, and give noteworthy experiences to medical care suppliers. In crisis circumstances or for people with intense medical issue, the fast correspondence worked with by 5G guarantees opportune mediations and further developed results.

Increased independent direction is a future pattern that highlights the cooperative connection between computer based intelligence frameworks and medical care experts. As man-made intelligence calculations become more refined, they can help medical care suppliers in pursuing complex choices overwhelmingly of information and producing proof based proposals.

Expanded direction is especially important in situations where the speed and exactness of information examination are basic. For example, in trauma centers or concentrated care units, simulated intelligence calculations can rapidly handle a large number of patient information, hailing possible issues, and helping medical services experts in settling on informed choices. This cooperative model guarantees that artificial intelligence supplements the ability of medical services suppliers, improving by and large quiet consideration.

Regardless of the promising future patterns of computer based intelligence driven wellbeing advances, moral contemplations stay principal. The mindful turn of events and organization of these advancements require cautious consideration regarding issues like information security, algorithmic predisposition, and straightforwardness. Administrative systems should develop to stay up with mechanical progressions, guaranteeing that computer based intelligence in medical care sticks to severe norms for security, adequacy, and moral use.

Information protection concerns, particularly with regards to wellbeing checking, require hearty shields. People should have command over their wellbeing information, with clear instruments for giving informed assent and quitting information sharing. Straightforwardness in how wellbeing information is gathered, put away, and used is fundamental for building and keeping up with trust between people, medical care suppliers, and innovation engineers.

Algorithmic predisposition is another moral thought that requires progressing watchfulness. One-sided calculations can prompt differences in medical care results, supporting existing imbalances. Engineers should focus on different and agent preparing datasets, consistently evaluate and reconsider algorithmic results, and impart straightforwardly about the impediments and potential predispositions inborn in computer based intelligence frameworks.

The fate of computer based intelligence driven wellbeing innovations likewise requires a pledge to tending to medical care inconsistencies. The advantages of these innovations ought to be open to different populaces, regardless of financial variables. Drives that elevate evenhanded admittance to innovation, give instruction on the most proficient method to utilize simulated intelligence empowered wellbeing checking apparatuses, and guarantee reasonableness are fundamental to forestall the compounding of existing wellbeing imbalances.

# Chapter 6

## Biofeedback and Neurotechnology

Biofeedback and neurotechnology address creative fields at the crossing point of medical services, innovation, and human physiology. These disciplines influence cutting edge innovations to screen, measure, and regulate physiological cycles, giving important experiences and mediations to wellbeing and prosperity. From stress the board to mental upgrade, biofeedback and neurotechnology offer a different scope of utilizations that keep on developing as how we might interpret the human mind and body extends.

Biofeedback, at its center, includes furnishing people with constant data about their physiological capabilities, empowering them to oversee these cycles. This data is ordinarily gathered through sensors that action different physiological boundaries, for example, pulse, skin conductance, muscle strain, and temperature. By picturing and understanding these physiological reactions, people can figure out how to control their physical processes, prompting further developed wellbeing results deliberately.

One normal use of biofeedback is in pressure the board. Ongoing pressure is a pervasive issue in present day culture, adding to different medical conditions. Biofeedback methods, for example, pulse changeability (HRV) preparing, intend to regulate the autonomic sensory system's reaction to stretch. HRV mirrors the fluctuation in the time stretches among pulses and is viewed as a sign of the body's capacity to adjust to pressure.

Biofeedback gadgets, frequently as wearable sensors or cell phone applications, guide people through practices that advance unwinding and lucidness in pulse designs. As clients take part in profound breathing or care rehearses, they get constant criticism on their HRV, assisting them with refining their procedures and accomplish a condition of physiological equilibrium. This further develops pressure versatility as well as has positive ramifications for cardiovascular wellbeing.

In the domain of torment the board, biofeedback has demonstrated powerful as a non-pharmacological mediation. People experiencing constant agony conditions, like headaches or fibromyalgia, can profit from biofeedback preparing to oversee physiological cycles related with torment discernment. By figuring out how to balance factors like muscle pressure and skin temperature, people might encounter a decrease in torment force and a better personal satisfaction.

Neurotechnology, then again, centers around advancements that point of interaction with the mind or the focal sensory system to screen, animate, or adjust brain movement. The headways in neurotechnology have opened up new wildernesses in grasping the cerebrum's intricacies and creating mediations for neurological issues and mental improvement.

One of the vital regions inside neurotechnology is neurofeedback, a particular type of biofeedback that spotlights on the mind's electrical movement, estimated through electroencephalography (EEG). Neurofeedback permits people to notice and direct their brainwave designs progressively, intending to streamline mental capability, oversee emotional wellness conditions, and upgrade in general prosperity.

With regards to emotional well-being, neurofeedback has shown guarantee in conditions like consideration shortfall/hyperactivity jumble (ADHD), nervousness, and sadness. People going through neurofeedback preparing participate in errands that require explicit brainwave designs related with concentration, unwinding, or close to home guideline. Through support components, for example, visual or hear-able prompts, clients figure out how to self-manage their mind action, possibly prompting upgrades in side effects.

Neurofeedback additionally holds likely applications in mental improvement. As how we might interpret the cerebrum's pliancy develops, neurotechnology mediations are being investigated to improve memory, consideration, and learning. Mind PC interfaces (BCIs) and neurostimulation methods, for example, transcranial attractive feeling (TMS) and transcranial direct current excitement (tDCS), are among the apparatuses utilized in this blossoming field.

BCIs empower direct correspondence between the cerebrum and outside gadgets, offering a pathway for people with engine disabilities to control prosthetic appendages or convey utilizing their contemplations. In the field of neurostimulation, TMS and tDCS include applying controlled electrical flows to the scalp, adjusting brain action and impacting mental cycles. These procedures are being explored for their true capacity in dealing with conditions like discouragement and improving mental execution in sound people.

The intermingling of biofeedback and neurotechnology addresses an all encompassing way to deal with upgrading human execution and prosperity. Consolidating physiological and brain estimations takes into consideration a more far reaching comprehension of how the psyche and body collaborate, opening up additional opportunities for customized intercessions and designated medical care techniques.

Combination of biofeedback and neurotechnology is clear in gadgets intended for both pressure the board and mental improvement. Wearable gadgets outfitted with EEG sensors, for instance, can give continuous criticism on both physiological and brain boundaries. People can follow their feelings of anxiety, pulse fluctuation, and brainwave designs all the while, acquiring a more nuanced comprehension of their general prosperity.

Besides, the advancement of computer generated reality (VR) applications in biofeedback and neurotechnology grandstands the potential for vivid encounters in helpful mediations. VR conditions can be custom-made to prompt explicit physiological or brain reactions, making controlled situations for biofeedback preparing or neurostimulation. This crossing point of innovation takes into account inventive ways to deal with address conditions like fears, PTSD, or neurological recovery.

Regardless of the promising utilizations of biofeedback and neurotechnology, moral contemplations should be painstakingly tended to. The assortment and understanding of physiological and brain information raise worries about individual protection and information security. Clear rules and administrative systems are fundamental to guarantee that delicate wellbeing data is taken care of capably, with informed assent and straightforward works on overseeing information use.

Also, the potential for abuse or unseen side-effects in mental improvement applications requires moral contemplations. Inquiries regarding reasonableness, value, and the expected cultural effect of inescapable mental improvement require smart investigation. As these advancements become more available, it is critical to think about the moral ramifications and lay out rules to forestall likely maltreatments or variations in access.

The job of medical care experts in the combination of biofeedback and neurotechnology is significant. While these advances engage people to play a functioning job in their wellbeing, direction from medical care suppliers is significant to guarantee protected and successful use. Medical care experts need to remain informed about the most recent headways, grasp the limits and likely dangers of these advances, and guide patients in their use.

Schooling and preparing programs for medical services experts ought to incorporate parts that acquaint them with biofeedback and neurotechnology. This improves how they might interpret these instruments as well as prepares them to incorporate these innovations into all encompassing patient consideration plans. Interdisciplinary cooperation between medical care suppliers, technologists, and scientists is fundamental for cultivate an exhaustive and moral way to deal with biofeedback and neurotechnology intercessions.

Looking forward, the eventual fate of biofeedback and neurotechnology holds invigorating conceivable outcomes. As these fields keep on propelling, the refinement of wearable gadgets, further developed availability of neuroimaging advancements, and the improvement of additional designated mediations are logical. The reconciliation of man-made reasoning and AI calculations further improves the capacity to examine complex physiological and brain information, giving customized bits of knowledge and intercessions.

In the clinical domain, biofeedback and neurotechnology may become standard parts of therapy plans for different circumstances, going from psychological wellness problems to ongoing agony the board. Customized medication approaches might integrate information from biofeedback and neurotechnology to tailor intercessions in view of a singular's remarkable physiological and brain reactions.

Research investigating the brain adaptability of the cerebrum and the potential for neurotechnology to improve mental capacities might prompt new intercessions for age-related mental deterioration or neurodegenerative issues. Cerebrum PC connection points might advance to offer more consistent and natural correspondence among people and outside gadgets, working on the personal satisfaction for those with engine impedances.

Likewise with any quickly propelling field, progressing research is fundamental to reveal the maximum capacity of biofeedback and neurotechnology. Longitudinal examinations, randomized controlled preliminaries, and cooperative endeavors across disciplines will add to the proof base supporting the adequacy and wellbeing of these mediations. Moral contemplations ought to stay at the front line, directing the mindful turn of events, arrangement, and combination of these advancements into medical services rehearses.

### 6.1 Introduction to biofeedback and its role in health monitoring

Biofeedback is a state of the art approach in medical services that engages people to oversee their physiological capabilities by giving constant data about real cycles. This strategy uses sensors to gauge different physiological boundaries, for example, pulse, skin conductance, muscle strain, and temperature. The ongoing criticism empowers people to turn out to be more mindful of their physiological reactions and figure out how to deliberately manage them, eventually adding to further developed wellbeing and prosperity.

The principal reason of biofeedback lies in the idea of self-guideline. By offering people quick input on their physiological states, biofeedback permits them to comprehend how their bodies answer various circumstances and boosts. This increased mindfulness turns into an integral asset for self-tweak, empowering people to oversee pressure, mitigate torment, and upgrade different parts of their wellbeing.

One of the vital utilizations of biofeedback is pressure the board. In the present quick moving and requesting world, constant pressure is an unavoidable issue that can unfavorably affect physical and emotional well-being. Biofeedback strategies, for example, pulse fluctuation (HRV) preparing, assume a pivotal part in pressure decrease. HRV, the variety in time spans between pulses, is a dependable mark of the body's capacity to adjust to pressure.

Biofeedback gadgets, frequently as wearable sensors or cell phone applications, guide people through practices intended to advance unwinding and soundness in pulse designs. Clients take part in profound breathing or care rehearses, and the biofeedback framework gives constant data on their HRV. This prompt input assists people with refining their pressure decrease methods, encouraging a condition of physiological equilibrium and strength to stressors.

Past pressure the executives, biofeedback is a significant device in torment the board. Persistent torment conditions, like headaches, fibromyalgia, or outer muscle torment, can altogether affect a singular's personal satisfaction. Biofeedback mediations center around assisting people with overseeing physiological cycles related with torment insight.

Through sensors that action muscle strain, skin temperature, or other important boundaries, people get continuous criticism on their substantial reactions to torment. Biofeedback preparing trains strategies to balance these physiological cycles, possibly prompting a decrease in torment power and an improvement in generally prosperity. The non-pharmacological nature of biofeedback makes it an engaging choice for those looking for options in contrast to conventional agony the board draws near.

Notwithstanding stress and torment the executives, biofeedback has found applications in different wellbeing spaces, including pulse guideline, nervousness issues, and gastrointestinal circumstances. Biofeedback procedures can help people in accomplishing explicit wellbeing objectives by advancing mindfulness and self-guideline of physiological cycles applicable to their circumstances.

The mix of biofeedback into wellbeing checking is especially remarkable with regards to wearable gadgets and advanced wellbeing innovations. Wearable sensors, frequently as smartwatches or wellness trackers, have become progressively complex in their capacity to screen physiological boundaries continuously. These gadgets influence biofeedback standards to give clients bits of knowledge into their wellbeing and prosperity.

For instance, wearable gadgets outfitted with pulse screens can offer nonstop input on pulse designs over the course of the day. People can see how their pulse answers various exercises, stressors, or times of rest. This data turns into an instrument for mindfulness, inciting clients to make way of life changes that emphatically influence their cardiovascular wellbeing.

Likewise, biofeedback standards are applied in wearable gadgets that track rest designs. Rest is a basic part of generally speaking wellbeing, and disturbances in rest can have flowing impacts on prosperity. Wearable gadgets with rest following capacities give clients input on their rest length, rest stages, and disturbances during the evening. Equipped with this data, people can settle on informed choices to further develop their rest cleanliness and generally rest quality.

The job of biofeedback in wellbeing checking reaches out past wearable gadgets to incorporate cell phone applications and computerized stages. Versatile applications outfitted with biofeedback elements can direct clients through unwinding works out, breathing strategies, or care works on, giving continuous criticism on their physiological reactions. This coordination of biofeedback into regular advances upgrades availability and convenience, permitting people to integrate self-guideline rehearses into their day to day schedules.

Also, the coming of telehealth and distant patient observing has extended the range of biofeedback intercessions. People can participate in biofeedback meetings with medical services experts from the solace of their homes, worked with by computerized stages that empower ongoing checking and criticism. This is especially advantageous for people with constant circumstances or those looking for progressing support for pressure the board and prosperity.

While biofeedback basically centers around the self-guideline of physiological boundaries, the field has developed to incorporate neurofeedback, a specific structure that focuses on the electrical movement of the cerebrum, estimated through electro-encephalography (EEG). Neurofeedback, otherwise called EEG biofeedback, offers people the chance to notice and tweak their brainwave designs progressively.

Neurofeedback is grounded in the possibility of brain adaptability, the mind's capacity to rearrange and adjust. By furnishing people with criticism on their brainwave designs, neurofeedback expects to work with positive changes in mental capability, close to home guideline, and by and large mind wellbeing. This area of biofeedback has acquired consideration for its possible applications in psychological well-being, mental upgrade, and neurological recovery.

In emotional wellness, neurofeedback has shown guarantee in conditions like consideration shortfall/hyperactivity jumble (ADHD), tension, and wretchedness. People going through neurofeedback preparing take part in assignments intended to evoke explicit brainwave designs related with concentration, unwinding, or close to home guideline. Through visual or hear-able signals that act as support, clients figure out how to self-direct their mind movement, possibly prompting upgrades in side effects.

Mental improvement is another region where neurofeedback holds potential. As how we might interpret the mind's pliancy develops, mediations that target explicit mental capabilities, like memory or consideration, are being investigated. Neurofeedback, joined with progressions in cerebrum PC interfaces (BCIs) and neurostimulation methods, offers additional opportunities for improving mental capacities in both solid people and those with mental disabilities.

Mind PC interfaces, which lay out an immediate correspondence pathway between the cerebrum and outer gadgets, have applications past neurofeedback. BCIs empower people with engine debilitations to control prosthetic appendages, convey through assistive advances, or connect with their surroundings utilizing their considerations. This creative utilization of biofeedback advancements exhibits their capability to upgrade the personal satisfaction for people with neurological circumstances.

Neurostimulation procedures, for example, transcranial attractive feeling (TMS) and transcranial direct current excitement (tDCS), are likewise essential for the advancing scene of biofeedback and neurotechnology. These harmless methods include applying controlled electrical flows or attractive fields to explicit region of the cerebrum, balancing brain movement and affecting mental cycles. Neurostimulation is being researched for its true capacity in dealing with conditions like wretchedness and upgrading mental execution.

The union of biofeedback and neurotechnology addresses a comprehensive way to deal with wellbeing observing and self-guideline. Wearable gadgets furnished with both physiological and brain sensors, joined with versatile applications and computerized stages, offer people a complete tool stash for observing and improving their wellbeing. The incorporation of man-made reasoning (simulated intelligence) and AI calculations further upgrades the capacities of these innovations, giving customized experiences and mediations in light of individual reactions.

As these innovations keep on progressing, moral contemplations stay central. The assortment and understanding of physiological and brain information raise worries about individual protection and information security. Clear rules and administrative systems are fundamental to guarantee that delicate wellbeing data is taken care of capably, with informed assent and straightforward works on administering information use.

Besides, the potential for abuse or unseen side-effects in mental upgrade applications requires moral contemplations. Inquiries concerning reasonableness, value, and the possible cultural effect of far reaching mental improvement require insightful investigation. As these advancements become more open, it is pivotal to think about the moral ramifications and lay out rules to forestall likely maltreatments or differences in access.

The job of medical care experts in the coordination of biofeedback and neurotechnology is significant. While these advances engage people to play a functioning job in their wellbeing, direction from medical care suppliers is significant to guarantee protected and viable use. Medical care experts need to remain informed about the most recent progressions, grasp the restrictions and likely dangers of these advancements, and guide patients in their usage.

Instruction and preparing programs for medical care experts ought to incorporate parts that acquaint them with biofeedback and neurotechnology. This upgrades how they might interpret these devices as well as prepares them to incorporate these advances into comprehensive patient consideration plans. Interdisciplinary joint effort between medical services suppliers, technologists, and specialists is crucial for cultivate an exhaustive and moral way to deal with biofeedback and neurotechnology intercessions.

Looking forward, the eventual fate of biofeedback and neurotechnology holds energizing prospects. As these fields keep on propelling, the refinement of wearable gadgets, further developed openness of neuroimaging innovations, and the advancement of additional designated mediations are logical. The combination of man-made reasoning and AI calculations further upgrades the capacity to dissect complex physiological and brain information, giving customized experiences and mediations.

In the clinical domain, biofeedback and neurotechnology may become standard parts of therapy plans for different circumstances, going from psychological wellbeing issues to ongoing agony the board. Customized medication approaches might integrate information from biofeedback and neurotechnology to tailor intercessions in light of a singular's extraordinary physiological and brain reactions.

Research investigating the brain adaptability of the cerebrum and the potential for neurotechnology to improve mental capacities might prompt new mediations for age-related mental deterioration or neurodegenerative issues. Cerebrum PC connection points might develop to offer more consistent and natural correspondence among people and outside gadgets, working on the personal satisfaction for those with engine debilitations.

Likewise with any quickly propelling field, continuous exploration is fundamental to reveal the maximum capacity of biofeedback and neurotechnology. Longitudinal investigations, randomized controlled preliminaries, and cooperative endeavors across disciplines will add to the proof base supporting the viability and security of these mediations. Moral contemplations ought to stay at the bleeding edge, directing the capable turn of events, arrangement, and joining of these advances into medical care rehearses.

## 6.2 Exploration of neurotechnology applications for stress reduction and mental well-being

Neurotechnology applications are progressively being investigated for their true capacity in pressure decrease and improving mental prosperity. As how we might interpret the cerebrum's intricacies extends, creative advancements are being created to adjust brain movement, advance unwinding, and add to in general mental health. From neurofeedback to cerebrum PC interfaces (BCIs), these headways offer new roads for customized intercessions and comprehensive ways to deal with emotional well-being.

Neurofeedback, a particular type of biofeedback, centers around observing and regulating the cerebrum's electrical action, normally estimated through electroencephalography (EEG). This innovation permits people to notice their own brainwave designs continuously and figure out how to self-manage these examples for explicit results. With regards to pressure decrease, neurofeedback has shown guarantee in preparing people to accomplish conditions of unwinding and worked on profound guideline.

The cycle includes putting EEG sensors on the scalp to catch brainwave movement. Through visual or hear-able input prompts, people are directed to deliver explicit brainwave designs related with unwinding and stress versatility. Over rehashed meetings, clients figure out how to perceive and regulate their cerebrum action, possibly prompting upgraded pressure survival strategies and worked on mental prosperity.

Neurofeedback's applications reach out past pressure decrease to incorporate circumstances like tension and consideration shortfall/hyperactivity jumble (ADHD). People with tension problems might profit from neurofeedback mediations intended to advance serenity and lessen hyperarousal states. Additionally, for people with ADHD, neurofeedback plans to upgrade consideration and self-guideline by building up unambiguous brainwave designs related with center.

Mind PC interfaces address one more outskirts in neurotechnology with applications for stress decrease and mental prosperity. BCIs lay out an immediate correspondence pathway between the cerebrum and outside gadgets, empowering people to control computerized interfaces or cooperate with their current circumstance utilizing their contemplations. With regards to pressure decrease, BCIs offer extraordinary opportunities for making customized intercessions in view of constant brain information.

For instance, BCIs can be used related to computer generated simulation (VR) conditions to make vivid and intuitive pressure decrease encounters. Clients, furnished with EEG sensors, can participate in VR situations intended to prompt conditions of unwinding and quiet. The BCI deciphers the client's brain movement, adjusting the VR climate continuously to improve the viability of stress decrease mediations. This powerful collaboration between the mind and innovation opens up creative pathways for custom-made mental wellbeing encounters.

Also, neurostimulation methods, for example, transcranial attractive excitement (TMS) and transcranial direct current feeling (tDCS), are being investigated for their true capacity in pressure decrease and state of mind improvement. These harmless techniques include applying controlled electrical flows or attractive fields to explicit region of the mind, regulating brain movement and affecting temperament related circuits.

TMS, for example, has been examined as a treatment for gloom by focusing on region of the cerebrum related with state of mind guideline. The thought is to actuate changes in brain action that lighten side effects of discouragement and work on in general mind-set. While these methods are still in the beginning phases of exploration, they address a promising road for neurotechnology applications in mental prosperity.

The personalization of neurotechnology intercessions for stress decrease is a critical area of investigation. Individual contrasts in brain reactions to stressors require approaches that think about the exceptional cerebrum marks of every individual. AI calculations and man-made reasoning (computer based intelligence) assume a urgent part in such manner, as they can dissect huge measures of neurophysiological information to distinguish examples and designer mediations in light of individual necessities.

The incorporation of neurotechnology with wearables and versatile applications further improves openness and convenience. Wearable gadgets furnished with EEG sensors or other neurophysiological observing abilities permit people to follow their feelings of anxiety continuously. Versatile applications can give criticism on pressure designs, guide clients through neurofeedback works out, and convey customized intercessions to help mental prosperity.

As these innovations advance, moral contemplations come to the front. Guaranteeing the protection and security of brain information is fundamental, as these information are exceptionally touchy and individual. Clear rules and administrative systems are important to oversee the mindful assortment, stockpiling, and utilization of neurophysiological data. Informed assent and straightforward practices are crucial for fabricate and keep up with trust among clients and innovation engineers.

Additionally, the potential for neurotechnology applications to impact mind-set and profound states brings up moral issues about the likely abuse or unseen side-effects. The capable turn of events and arrangement of these advances require cautious thought of the cultural effect, likely dangers, and evenhanded admittance to mediations. Moral rules ought to be laid out to forestall abberations in access and guarantee that the advantages of neurotechnology are available to assorted populaces.

The job of medical services experts in the investigation of neurotechnology applications for stress decrease is significant. While these advancements engage people to play a functioning job in dealing with their psychological prosperity, direction from medical services suppliers is fundamental to guarantee protected and viable use. Medical services experts need to remain informed about the most recent headways, grasp the restrictions and expected dangers of these advancements, and guide patients in their use.

Schooling and preparing programs for medical services experts ought to incorporate parts that acclimate them with neurotechnology applications and their suggestions for emotional well-being. Interdisciplinary cooperation between medical care suppliers, neuroscientists, technologists, and ethicists is fundamental to explore the mind boggling scene of neurotechnology in pressure decrease.

Looking forward, the future of neurotechnology applications for stress decrease holds energizing prospects. As how we might interpret the cerebrum proceeds to advance, and innovation turns out to be more modern, customized mediations custom-made to individual brain reactions might become typical. Wearable gadgets may flawlessly incorporate neurophysiological observing into regular daily existence, giving constant criticism and intercessions to help mental prosperity.

Headways in computer based intelligence and AI will probably assume a focal part in refining the personalization of neurotechnology mediations. These advancements can examine complex brain information designs, distinguish individual pressure reaction profiles, and powerfully change mediations progressively. The collaboration between neurotechnology, wearables, and computer based intelligence opens up new boondocks in psychological wellness support.

### 6.3 Potential future developments in these fields

The fields of biofeedback and neurotechnology are ready for huge headways, preparing for groundbreaking improvements that could reshape the scene of medical care and prosperity. Planning ahead, a few expected developments and forward leaps are not too far off, offering energizing opportunities for customized medication, upgraded mental capacities, and novel intercessions.

One potential future advancement lies in the assembly of biofeedback and neurotechnology, making coordinated frameworks that influence both physiological and brain information. Wearable gadgets outfitted with cutting edge sensors could consistently screen a more extensive scope of physiological boundaries, including pulse, skin conductance, and brainwave designs estimated through EEG. This combination would give clients a more thorough comprehension of their brain body association, taking into consideration designated mediations that address both physiological and brain parts of wellbeing.

The refinement of wearable gadgets is one more road for future turn of events.

As innovation keeps on propelling, wearables might turn out to be more complex, conservative, and able to do constant checking. Scaled down sensors with further developed precision could offer clients consistent bits of knowledge into their well-being, empowering proactive measures for pressure the executives, customized wellness plans, and early location of medical problems. The client experience might turn out to be more consistent, adding to the joining of biofeedback and neurotechnology into regular daily existence.

The use of man-made consciousness (artificial intelligence) and AI calculations in biofeedback and neurotechnology is a promising wilderness for future turn of events. These innovations can dissect huge datasets, recognizing complicated examples and relationships that may not be clear through conventional strategies. In biofeedback, artificial intelligence could upgrade the personalization of mediations by progressively adjusting to a person's changing physiological reactions. In neurotechnology, AI calculations could advance neurofeedback conventions in view of ongoing brain information, prompting more proficient and compelling mediations.

In the domain of neurotechnology, mind PC interfaces (BCIs) are probably going to go through critical progressions. Improved BCI innovation could offer people more natural and consistent command over outer gadgets, opening up additional opportunities for assistive advancements and correspondence for people with engine debilitations. Further developed BCI frameworks may likewise track down applications in neurorehabilitation, working with recuperation from neurological wounds and problems.

The improvement of shut circle neurostimulation frameworks addresses another thrilling road. These frameworks would progressively change feeling boundaries in light of continuous brain criticism, improving the adequacy of neurostimulation mediations. Shut circle neurostimulation holds guarantee in treating conditions like discouragement, persistent agony, and neurological problems by fitting mediations to individual brain reactions, possibly further developing results and decreasing secondary effects.

Customized medication approaches utilizing biofeedback and neurotechnology may turn out to be more ordinary. The mix of hereditary, way of life, and physiological/brain information could empower medical care suppliers to make profoundly individualized therapy plans. For instance, joining hereditary data with biofeedback information might assist with foreseeing a singular's vulnerability to push related conditions, taking into account precautionary intercessions custom-made to their remarkable organic cosmetics.

Progressions in distant patient observing and telehealth are supposed to assume a huge part coming soon for these fields. The capacity to remotely screen physiological and brain boundaries, combined with continuous criticism and intercessions, could alter how medical services is conveyed. Patients with constant circumstances or those going through neurofeedback preparing could profit from the accommodation and availability of remote observing, upgrading congruity of care and working on tolerant results.

The moral contemplations encompassing these potential improvements can't be ignored. As biofeedback and neurotechnology become more incorporated into medical care, information protection, security, and informed assent should be focused on. Clear rules and guidelines ought to be laid out to guarantee the dependable and moral utilization of delicate wellbeing data. Furthermore, resolving issues of algorithmic predisposition and guaranteeing fair admittance to these advancements are fundamental to forestall differences in medical care results.

Schooling and preparing programs for medical services experts should advance to consolidate these arising innovations. As biofeedback and neurotechnology become more indispensable to medical care rehearses, medical services suppliers should be outfitted with the information and abilities to really explore these fields. Interdisciplinary coordinated effort between medical services experts, technologists, ethicists, and analysts will be pivotal to creating moral and compelling ways to deal with execution.

# Chapter 7

## Smart Home Health Systems

Savvy home wellbeing frameworks address a groundbreaking convergence of innovation and medical care, meaning to improve the prosperity of people inside the solace of their homes. These frameworks influence the most recent headways in brilliant gadgets, sensors, man-made consciousness (artificial intelligence), and availability to make a coordinated biological system that screens wellbeing measurements, upholds clinical administration, and works with proactive medical services mediations. As the world wrestles with a maturing populace, the rising pervasiveness of persistent sicknesses, and the interest for more customized medical care arrangements, brilliant home wellbeing frameworks arise as a promising road for further developing medical care results and enabling people to play a functioning job in dealing with their wellbeing.

One of the primary parts of savvy home wellbeing frameworks is distant wellbeing checking. Wearable gadgets furnished with sensors, for example, smartwatches or wellness trackers, gather continuous information on essential signs, active work, and other wellbeing related measurements. These gadgets consistently associate with the more extensive brilliant home environment, considering ceaseless wellbeing observing without expecting people to participate in information assortment effectively. This ability is especially valuable for people with persistent circumstances, more established grown-ups, or those recuperating from operations, as it empowers medical services suppliers to remotely screen their wellbeing status and intercede expeditiously if necessary.

Notwithstanding wearables, brilliant home wellbeing frameworks frequently consolidate different sensors inserted inside the residing climate. For instance, brilliant scales, circulatory strain screens, and glucose meters can send information straightforwardly to the focal wellbeing observing stage. Movement sensors and cameras might be decisively positioned to distinguish changes in development designs or recognize possible falls, particularly significant for more seasoned grown-ups or people with portability issues. These encompassing sensors work synergistically to make an exhaustive image of a singular's wellbeing and way of life, working with early recognition of medical problems and convenient intercession.

The joining of computer based intelligence and AI calculations is a critical driver in the viability of brilliant home wellbeing frameworks. These calculations break down the immense measure of wellbeing information created by wearable gadgets and encompassing sensors, separating significant experiences and distinguishing designs that might slip by everyone's notice by customary medical services draws near. Computer based intelligence controlled prescient examination can expect potential medical problems in view of changes in designs, considering proactive mediations and customized medical care plans. For instance, AI calculations can break down a blend of information, for example, rest designs, action levels, and important bodily functions, to foresee the probability of a wellbeing disintegration or the beginning of a persistent condition.

Prescription administration is one more basic part of savvy home wellbeing frameworks. These frameworks can integrate brilliant pill distributors that give drug updates, apportion the right measurement at planned times, and send cautions to the two people and medical services suppliers assuming portions are missed. Mix with electronic wellbeing records (EHRs) takes into account consistent correspondence between the brilliant home wellbeing framework and medical care experts, guaranteeing that drug adherence is firmly observed. This usefulness is particularly important for people with constant circumstances that require severe prescription regimens.

Besides, shrewd home wellbeing frameworks can upgrade the providing care insight for both expert parental figures and relatives. Remote checking capacities furnish parental figures with constant experiences into the wellbeing status and exercises of their patients or friends and family. This works with early identification of medical problems as well as permits guardians to offer opportune help and mediations. On account of more seasoned grown-ups or people with mental debilitations, savvy home frameworks can incorporate elements like robotized updates for day to day undertakings, crisis reaction frameworks, and, surprisingly, virtual friendship through voice-actuated partners.

Voice-actuated remote helpers, like Amazon's Alexa or Google Aide, are necessary parts of brilliant home wellbeing frameworks. These partners can be modified to give drug updates, answer wellbeing related questions, and even participate in intelligent wellbeing training. People can utilize voice orders to actually take a look at their wellbeing measurements, plan arrangements, or get customized wellbeing guidance. The conversational idea of menial helpers makes them especially available for people of changing ages and innovative education, encouraging client commitment and adherence to wellbeing the executives plans.

Protection and security are principal contemplations in the turn of events and arrangement of savvy home wellbeing frameworks. As these frameworks manage touchy wellbeing information, strong encryption, validation instruments, and consistence with medical care information insurance guidelines are fundamental. Producers and designers should focus on the security of both the gadgets and the information they gather to impart trust in clients and medical services suppliers. Clear correspondence about information utilization strategies, informed assent, and straightforward works on in regards to information imparting to medical services experts are pivotal to tending to security concerns.

Interoperability is one more test that savvy home wellbeing frameworks need to defeat for boundless reception and viability. As the environment of gadgets and stages keeps on extending, guaranteeing consistent correspondence between various brands and kinds of gadgets is fundamental. Normalized conventions and open structures can work with interoperability, permitting people to pick gadgets that best suit their requirements while guaranteeing similarity with the more extensive shrewd home wellbeing framework.

The coordination of telehealth administrations inside savvy home wellbeing frameworks further improves their abilities. Video meetings, remote observing, and virtual wellbeing instructing meetings can be flawlessly coordinated into the general wellbeing the board plan. This is particularly significant for people with portability limits, those in remote or underserved regions, or people who favor the accommodation of virtual medical care associations. Telehealth inside brilliant home frameworks gives an all encompassing way to deal with medical services, joining remote checking, information driven experiences, and direct correspondence with medical services experts.

The potential for shrewd home wellbeing frameworks reaches out past the administration of constant circumstances to proactive wellbeing and health advancement. These frameworks can consolidate elements like customized wellness schedules, nourishment direction, and emotional well-being support. By dissecting individual wellbeing information, brilliant home frameworks can give fitted proposals to actual work, rest cleanliness, and stress the board. This comprehensive way to deal with wellbeing and wellbeing lines up with the shift towards preventive medical care and enables people to pursue informed way of life decisions.

As shrewd home wellbeing frameworks keep on advancing, progressing innovative work are fundamental to refine their abilities and address arising difficulties. Long haul studies evaluating the adequacy of these frameworks in further developing wellbeing results, decreasing medical care costs, and improving the personal satisfaction are significant for building proof based rehearses. Coordinated efforts between innovation designers, medical care suppliers, specialists, and administrative bodies are instrumental in forming the future direction of savvy home wellbeing frameworks.

### 7.1 Overview of integrated smart home devices for health monitoring

Coordinated savvy home gadgets for wellbeing observing are at the front of the transformation in customized medical care. This imaginative biological system joins state of the art innovations, like sensors, man-made brainpower (computer based intelligence), and network, to make a consistent and exhaustive way to deal with wellbeing the executives inside the home climate. The reconciliation of these gadgets permits people to screen fundamental wellbeing measurements, get constant bits of knowledge, and even access virtual medical care administrations, changing how wellbeing is checked and made due.

Wearable gadgets, for example, smartwatches and wellness trackers, structure the central layer of coordinated shrewd home wellbeing observing. These gadgets are furnished with a variety of sensors, including pulse screens, accelerometers, and GPS, empowering constant following of actual work, rest designs, and cardiovascular wellbeing. Wearables flawlessly interface with other shrewd home gadgets, making an all encompassing wellbeing observing biological system.

The ongoing information gathered by wearables fills in as an establishment for customized wellbeing bits of knowledge. For instance, consistent pulse checking can offer bits of knowledge into feelings of anxiety, practice power, and by and large cardiovascular wellbeing. Rest following gives data about rest term, rest stages, and interruptions, offering a thorough comprehension of one's rest quality. These experiences engage people to settle on informed conclusions about their way of life, work-out schedules, and rest cleanliness, adding to generally speaking wellbeing and prosperity.

Encompassing sensors decisively positioned inside the home climate supplement wearables, making a more far reaching wellbeing checking framework. Brilliant scales, circulatory strain screens, and glucose meters flawlessly send information to the focal wellbeing checking stage. This takes into consideration the nonstop checking of indispensable wellbeing measurements without the requirement for manual info, guaranteeing a more precise and continuous portrayal of a singular's wellbeing status.

Movement sensors and cameras inside the home climate assume a pivotal part in wellbeing observing, particularly for more seasoned grown-ups or people with versatility issues. These sensors can distinguish changes in development designs, recognize likely falls, and give alarms to parental figures or crisis administrations when required. The combination of visual information from cameras considers extra setting, working with remote observing and opportune mediations.

The reconciliation of computerized reasoning and AI calculations lifts the capacities of savvy home wellbeing checking. These calculations investigate the tremendous measure of wellbeing information produced by wearables and encompassing sensors, distinguishing examples and relationships that might slip through the cracks by customary medical services draws near. Artificial intelligence driven prescient examination can expect potential medical problems in light of changes in designs, empowering proactive mediations and customized medical care plans.

Prescription administration is a basic part of wellbeing observing, particularly for people with constant circumstances. Brilliant pill containers with network to the focal wellbeing observing stage give drug updates, administer the right measurement at planned times, and send cautions to people and medical services suppliers assuming that dosages are missed. This component guarantees that drug adherence is firmly checked and takes into consideration opportune intercessions to resolve any issues.

Voice-actuated remote helpers, like Amazon's Alexa or Google Aide, are necessary parts of coordinated brilliant home wellbeing checking. These menial helpers can be modified to give drug updates, answer wellbeing related questions, and even participate in intelligent wellbeing training. People can utilize voice orders to actually take a look at their wellbeing measurements, plan arrangements, or get customized wellbeing exhortation, making wellbeing the board open and easy to use.

Protection and security contemplations are vital in the turn of events and arrangement of coordinated shrewd home wellbeing checking. As these frameworks handle touchy wellbeing information, strong encryption, confirmation components, and consistence with medical services information security guidelines are fundamental. Makers and engineers should focus on the security of both the gadgets and the information they gather to impart trust in clients and medical services suppliers. Clear correspondence about information utilization arrangements, informed assent, and straightforward works on in regards to information imparting to medical services experts are significant to tending to protection concerns.

Interoperability is a key test that coordinated savvy home wellbeing checking frameworks need to defeat for far reaching reception and viability. With a large number of gadgets and stages accessible, guaranteeing consistent correspondence between various brands and sorts of gadgets is fundamental. Normalized conventions and open designs can work with interoperability, permitting people to pick gadgets that best suit their necessities while guaranteeing similarity with the more extensive wellbeing observing framework.

The reconciliation of telehealth administrations inside savvy home wellbeing checking frameworks further upgrades their capacities. Video conferences, remote checking, and virtual wellbeing training meetings can be flawlessly incorporated into the general wellbeing the board plan. This is particularly significant for people with versatility limits, those in remote or underserved regions, or people who lean toward the accommodation of virtual medical care collaborations. Telehealth inside shrewd home frameworks gives an all encompassing way to deal with medical services, joining remote checking, information driven experiences, and direct correspondence with medical care experts.

The potential for coordinated savvy home wellbeing checking reaches out past the administration of constant circumstances to proactive wellbeing and health advancement. These frameworks can consolidate elements like customized wellness schedules, nourishment direction, and psychological well-being support. By investigating individual wellbeing information, brilliant home frameworks can give fitted suggestions to actual work, rest cleanliness, and stress the executives. This comprehensive way to deal with wellbeing and wellbeing lines up with the shift towards preventive medical services and engages people to settle on informed way of life decisions.

As incorporated brilliant home wellbeing checking frameworks keep on advancing, progressing innovative work are fundamental to refine their capacities and address arising difficulties. Long haul studies surveying the viability of these frameworks in further developing wellbeing results, diminishing medical services costs, and upgrading the personal satisfaction are urgent for building proof based rehearses. Coordinated efforts between innovation engineers, medical care suppliers, scientists, and administrative bodies are instrumental in molding the future direction of coordinated shrewd home wellbeing checking.

## 7.2 Discussion on how IoT (Internet of Things) contributes to a connected health ecosystem

The Web of Things (IoT) has arisen as a critical power in changing medical services, leading to an associated wellbeing biological system that holds the commitment of worked on persistent results, improved productivity, and a shift towards proactive and customized medical services.

The reconciliation of IoT in medical services has empowered the consistent network of gadgets, sensors, and frameworks, making an organization that works with continuous information trade, remote checking, and information driven navigation. This conversation dives into how IoT adds to the associated wellbeing environment, investigating the multi-layered influence on persistent consideration, medical services conveyance, and the general medical services scene.

### Distant Patient Observing and Wearables:

One of the vital commitments of IoT to the associated wellbeing biological system is in far off quiet observing. Wearable gadgets installed with sensors, for example, smartwatches and wellness trackers, permit people to constantly follow imperative signs, actual work, and other wellbeing measurements. These wearables communicate ongoing information to medical services suppliers, making a persistent transfer of data that empowers remote checking. This capacity is especially vital for patients with persistent circumstances, postoperative consideration, or those requiring progressing wellbeing the board.

Through IoT-empowered wearables, medical services suppliers can get to an extensive arrangement of patient information, including pulse, rest examples, and movement levels. This constant observing works with early discovery of irregularities, empowering ideal mediations and decreasing the requirement for successive in-person visits. Patients benefit from the comfort of remote observing, as it permits them to remain associated with their medical care suppliers while keeping up with their everyday schedules.

### Surrounding and Locally situated Observing:

IoT expands its effect past wearable gadgets to incorporate encompassing and locally situated checking arrangements. Shrewd home gadgets, outfitted with sensors, empower the persistent observing of a singular's residing climate. For instance, shrewd scales, circulatory strain screens, and glucose meters flawlessly coordinate with the IoT environment, sending wellbeing information straightforwardly to medical services suppliers. This encompassing checking makes a more comprehensive perspective on a singular's wellbeing, offering bits of knowledge into way of life factors that might influence their prosperity.

With regards to maturing populaces and people with constant circumstances, IoT-empowered locally established checking gives a proactive way to deal with medical care. Movement sensors and cameras decisively positioned inside the home climate can distinguish changes in development designs, recognize possible falls, and proposition significant data for parental figures and medical care suppliers. This improves security as well as adds to the general administration of constant circumstances by giving a ceaseless stream of significant wellbeing information.

**Information Driven Experiences and Prescient Examination:**

The tremendous measure of information created by IoT gadgets shapes the establishment for information driven experiences and prescient examination. Simulated intelligence and AI calculations break down this information, distinguishing examples, connections, and patterns that may not be clear through conventional techniques. In the associated wellbeing environment, these experiences engage medical services suppliers to settle on informed choices, tailor therapy designs, and expect potential medical problems.

For example, prescient examination can use IoT information to expect illness intensifications or difficulties for patients with constant circumstances. By dissecting patterns in essential signs, medicine adherence, and other significant boundaries, medical services suppliers can mediate proactively, possibly forestalling hospitalizations or intense episodes. This prescient capacity lines up with the shift towards preventive medical services, taking into consideration a more proactive and customized way to deal with patient consideration.

**Medicine Adherence and Brilliant Pill Allocators:**

IoT adds to medicine the board through the combination of brilliant pill containers. These gadgets, associated with the IoT environment, offer highlights like drug updates, administering the right dose at booked times, and sending cautions to the two people and medical services suppliers assuming dosages are missed. Drug adherence is a basic calculate overseeing ongoing circumstances, and IoT-empowered arrangements improve the checking and backing of people in sticking to their prescription regimens.

Via consistently incorporating with electronic wellbeing records (EHRs) and the more extensive associated wellbeing biological system, savvy pill distributors give a thorough perspective taking drugs adherence. This data is important for medical care suppliers in changing therapy plans, surveying the viability of meds, and resolving potential issues connected with non-adherence. IoT-empowered drug the executives encourages a cooperative methodology among people and their medical care groups, further developing generally wellbeing results.

**Telehealth Administrations and Virtual Medical care:**

IoT assumes a urgent part in the extension of telehealth administrations inside the associated wellbeing biological system. The availability of gadgets, wearables, and encompassing sensors empowers people to take part in virtual medical care conferences, remote observing, and telehealth mediations. Video discussions, worked with by IoT network, overcome any barrier between medical services suppliers and patients, particularly for those in remote or underserved regions.

The mix of telehealth administrations inside the IoT environment considers a consistent progression of wellbeing information among people and medical care suppliers.

This virtual network improves availability to medical care administrations, advances early intercessions, and supports continuous administration of ailments. Telehealth, empowered by IoT, adds to a patient-driven way to deal with medical care, where people can get to medical services benefits helpfully and get opportune help.

**Difficulties and Contemplations:**

While IoT carries significant advantages to the associated wellbeing environment, it likewise presents difficulties and contemplations. Protection and security are central worries, given the delicate idea of wellbeing information. Guaranteeing hearty encryption, validation systems, and consistence with medical services information insurance guidelines are urgent. Clear correspondence about information use strategies, informed assent, and straightforward works on in regards to information imparting to medical services experts are crucial for address security concerns.

Interoperability stays a test in the consistent reconciliation of different IoT gadgets and stages. Normalized conventions and open structures are expected to work with interoperability, permitting people to pick gadgets that suit their necessities while guaranteeing similarity with the more extensive associated wellbeing framework. Furthermore, progressing innovative work are fundamental to refine the abilities of IoT in medical services, address arising difficulties, and assemble proof based rehearses.

**7.3 Examples of smart home technologies for monitoring nutrition, air quality, and overall well-being**

Savvy home advances have quickly developed, offering imaginative answers for screen different parts of day to day existence, including nourishment, air quality, and in general prosperity. These advancements influence sensors, network, and information investigation to give ongoing bits of knowledge, enabling people to arrive at informed conclusions about their wellbeing and way of life. In this conversation, we investigate instances of savvy home advancements in these spaces, displaying how they add to an all encompassing way to deal with prosperity inside the home climate.

1. **Nourishment Observing:**

1. **Brilliant Fridges and Storage spaces:**

    Brilliant fridges and storage spaces are furnished with sensors and cameras that permit people to monitor their food stock progressively.

    These gadgets can identify and log the things present, their termination dates, and, surprisingly, give thoughts for recipes in view of accessible fixings. This assists in diminishing food with squandering as well as advances better dietary patterns by empowering people to utilize new fixings.

2. **Shrewd Kitchen Machines:**

    IoT-empowered kitchen machines, like brilliant blenders, scales, and broilers, give help with planning nutritious dinners. These gadgets can give segment control thoughts, track the wholesome substance of fixings, and even suggest recipes in view of dietary inclinations or limitations. Via flawlessly coordinating with wellbeing related applications, these machines add to a more cognizant and informed way to deal with nourishment.

3. **Supplement Following Applications and Shrewd Utensils:**

Versatile applications that attention on supplement following can adjust with brilliant utensils outfitted with sensors. These utensils can gauge segment measures and give continuous input on wholesome substance. This mix of applications and utensils permits people to screen their calorie consumption, track macronutrients, and pursue better food decisions.

**2. Air Quality Observing:**

1. **Savvy Air Purifiers:**
   Savvy air purifiers consolidate sensors to gauge air quality progressively. These gadgets can recognize poisons, allergens, and particulate matter in the air. With IoT availability, they can be controlled from a distance, and clients get notices about changes in air quality. This is especially useful for people with respiratory circumstances or sensitivities, empowering them to establish a better indoor climate.

2. **Savvy Indoor regulators and air conditioning Frameworks:**
   IoT-empowered indoor regulators and warming, ventilation, and cooling (air conditioning) frameworks add to air quality by directing temperature and moistness levels. These gadgets can be modified to keep up with ideal circumstances, forestalling the development of shape and decreasing the presence of airborne allergens. A few high level frameworks even coordinate air quality sensors to consequently change settings in view of ongoing estimations.

3. **Air Quality Checking Stations:**

Devoted air quality observing stations, frequently positioned in living regions, consistently measure different boundaries, for example, carbon dioxide levels, unstable natural mixtures (VOCs), and particulate matter. These stations give definite experiences into the general air quality inside the home. Reconciliation with savvy home frameworks permits clients to get alarms and make moves to further develop air quality when required.

**3. In general Prosperity Observing:**

1. **Wearable Wellbeing Trackers:**
   Wearable gadgets, for example, smartwatches and wellness trackers, stretch out past observing active work. They currently incorporate highlights for following rest designs, feelings of anxiety, and generally speaking prosperity. These wearables use sensors to quantify pulse fluctuation, skin conductance, and rest quality. The information gathered gives people an all encompassing perspective on

their prosperity and helps in making way of life changes for further developed wellbeing.

2. **Brilliant Beds and Sleeping pads:**
High level rest innovation incorporates brilliant beds and beddings that screen rest designs, body developments, and, surprisingly, respiratory rate. These gadgets give experiences into the nature of rest, recognizing times of fretfulness or potential rest unsettling influences. Coordinating with other savvy home frameworks, they can add to establishing an ideal rest climate by changing elements like lighting and temperature.

3. **Voice-Enacted Remote helpers for Prosperity:**

Voice-enacted menial helpers, similar to Amazon's Alexa or Google Collaborator, assume a part in general prosperity. These colleagues can give directed reflection meetings, offer wellbeing related data, and even recommend unwinding procedures. By incorporating with other shrewd home gadgets, they add to establishing a quieting climate, changing lighting, or playing mitigating music in view of client inclinations.

**4. Integrative Shrewd Home Environments:**

1. **Incorporated Brilliant Home Center points:**
Incorporated brilliant home center points, frequently fueled by artificial intelligence, act as the mind of the associated home. These center points coordinate information from different sensors and gadgets, giving a unified stage to checking nourishment, air quality, and in general prosperity. Clients can get to exhaustive bits of knowledge and control various parts of their home climate through a solitary connection point.

2. **Wellbeing Dashboards and Applications:**

Wellbeing dashboards and applications total information from various brilliant home gadgets, offering a combined perspective on sustenance, air quality, and in general prosperity. These applications frequently influence AI calculations to give customized proposals in view of the gathered information. Clients can follow patterns, put forth wellbeing objectives, and get noteworthy experiences to upgrade their prosperity.

**Difficulties and Contemplations:**
While brilliant home advances bring various advantages, there are provokes and contemplations to address. Protection and information security are principal, particularly while managing touchy wellbeing data. Producers should carry out vigorous safety efforts, encryption, and client validation to safeguard people's information. Straightforward information utilization approaches and clear assent components are fundamental for construct trust among clients.

Interoperability stays a test in making consistent reconciliations between various shrewd home gadgets and stages. Normalized conventions and open structures can work with interoperability, guaranteeing that clients can pick gadgets that suit their requirements while as yet being viable with the more extensive shrewd home environment.

**7.4 Challenges and considerations in adopting smart home health systems**

The reception of savvy home wellbeing frameworks presents a change in outlook in medical care conveyance, promising customized and helpful answers for observing and overseeing wellbeing inside the home climate. Notwithstanding, close by the possible advantages, there are huge difficulties and contemplations that should be addressed to guarantee the inescapable acknowledgment, viability, and moral utilization of these advancements. This conversation investigates the vital difficulties and contemplations in embracing shrewd home wellbeing frameworks.

1. **Protection and Information Security:**

   One of the premier worries in the reception of savvy home wellbeing frameworks is the protection and security of delicate wellbeing information. These frameworks gather and interaction an abundance of individual data, including wellbeing measurements, prescription adherence, and way of life designs. Guaranteeing strong encryption, secure information stockpiling, and assurance against unapproved access are basic to shield people's protection. Finding some kind of harmony between information convenience for medical services suppliers and saving client security is a sensitive test that requires severe administrative structures and industry principles.

2. **Interoperability and Normalization:**

   The savvy home wellbeing biological system is huge, with a large number of gadgets and stages created by various makers. Interoperability, or the consistent correspondence between different gadgets and frameworks, is a basic test. The absence of normalized conventions and open models thwarts the joining of different gadgets.

   Accomplishing interoperability is fundamental to permit clients the adaptability to pick gadgets that suit their requirements while guaranteeing similarity with the more extensive wellbeing checking framework. Industry cooperation and the foundation of normal guidelines are significant stages in beating this test.

3. **Client Acknowledgment and Convenience:**

   The effective reception of brilliant home wellbeing frameworks relies upon client acknowledgment and usability. People, particularly more seasoned grown-ups or those with restricted specialized capability, may find it trying to explore complex connection points or figure out the functionalities of different gadgets. Planning instinctive UIs, giving clear guidelines, and offering easy to use support are crucial for improve client acknowledgment. Guaranteeing that these advancements flawlessly coordinate into day to day existence without causing extra pressure is fundamental for supported commitment.

4. **Moral Contemplations and Informed Assent:**
   The moral ramifications of brilliant home wellbeing frameworks reach out past information protection. Issues like informed assent, straightforwardness, and mindful utilization of information are basic. Clients should be all around informed about how their wellbeing information will be gathered, put away, and shared. Straightforward information use arrangements, clear assent components, and the capacity for clients to control and repudiate authorizations are vital for address moral worries. Finding some kind of harmony between the advantages of information driven medical services and regarding individual independence is essential for cultivating trust.

5. **Unwavering quality and Precision of Wellbeing Information:**
   The unwavering quality and precision of wellbeing information created by savvy home gadgets are fundamental for compelling medical services mediations. Wearable gadgets, sensors, and observing apparatuses should give exact estimations and reliable information after some time. Fluctuation or errors in information might prompt wrong wellbeing appraisals, possibly compromising patient consideration. Thorough testing, approval cycles, and adherence to laid out quality norms are fundamental to guarantee the dependability of wellbeing information gathered by these gadgets.

6. **Mix with Conventional Medical care Frameworks:**
   Brilliant home wellbeing frameworks must flawlessly incorporate with customary medical care foundation, including electronic wellbeing records (EHRs) and medical care supplier work processes. The absence of coordination might bring about divided medical services conveyance, with information dwelling in storehouses that frustrate thorough patient consideration.
   Creating normalized interfaces and advancing interoperability between brilliant home gadgets and existing medical care frameworks are essential moves toward address this test. Medical care suppliers ought to have the option to get to and integrate significant savvy home information into their dynamic cycles.

7. **Cost and Openness:**
   The underlying expense of procuring and executing savvy home wellbeing frameworks can be a huge hindrance to reception. While the drawn out benefits, like decreased hospitalizations and further developed wellbeing results, may legitimize the venture, the forthright costs might restrict availability, especially for underserved populaces. Guaranteeing reasonableness and investigating roads for monetary help or protection inclusion can assist with alleviating this test. Finding some kind of harmony between cost-viability and the expected long haul reserve funds in medical services uses is fundamental for the far reaching reception of these advancements.

8. **Specialized Difficulties and Framework Intricacy:**
   The specialized intricacy of brilliant home wellbeing frameworks presents difficulties connected with gadget interoperability, programming updates, and

framework upkeep. Clients might confront hardships in setting up gadgets, investigating specialized issues, or staying aware of programming overhauls. Offering hearty specialized help, easy to understand manuals, and planning frameworks that limit specialized errors are urgent contemplations to improve the general client experience and lessen the weight on people.

9. **Administrative and Legitimate Systems:**
   The administrative scene for savvy home wellbeing frameworks is developing, and there is a requirement for clear rules and norms. Administrative bodies should resolve issues connected with information security, protection, and the moral utilization of wellbeing information. Laying out structures that guarantee consistence with medical services guidelines, assurance of patient freedoms, and responsibility for framework engineers is pivotal for building trust among clients and medical services experts.

10. **Constant Exploration and Proof Based Practices:**

As brilliant home wellbeing frameworks keep on developing, there is a requirement for ceaseless exploration to survey their viability, influence on wellbeing results, and likely dangers. Proof based practices ought to direct the turn of events and sending of these advancements. Long haul studies, clinical preliminaries, and cooperation between specialists, medical services suppliers, and innovation engineers are vital for construct a hearty information base and illuminate best practices in the field.

# Chapter 8

### Advancements in Vital Sign Monitoring

Progressions in essential sign observing play had a groundbreaking impact in medical services, offering new aspects in quiet consideration, remote checking, and early location of medical problems. As innovation keeps on developing, the mix of creative sensors, wearable gadgets, man-made brainpower (simulated intelligence), and network has prompted a change in outlook in how medical services experts and people track and decipher imperative signs. This conversation investigates the new headways in imperative sign observing, the effect on tolerant results, and the more extensive ramifications for the fate of medical services.

1. **Wearable Gadgets for Ceaseless Checking:**
   Wearable gadgets have arisen as integral assets for constant essential sign observing, giving continuous information on key physiological boundaries. Smartwatches, wellness trackers, and other wearable sensors are furnished with innovations, for example, photoplethysmography (PPG) and accelerometers to quantify pulse, blood oxygen levels, and actual work. Ceaseless observing takes into consideration an exhaustive comprehension of a singular's wellbeing past the requirements of inconsistent center visits.

   The mix of wearables into day to day existence empowers people to proactively deal with their wellbeing. Ceaseless checking of pulse changeability, for instance, can offer bits of knowledge into feelings of anxiety and by and large cardiovascular wellbeing. Wearables outfitted with ECG capacities give a more definite examination of heart musicality, supporting the early recognition of arrhythmias. These headways engage people to assume responsibility for their prosperity by giving noteworthy experiences and working with early mediations.

2. **Distant Patient Checking Frameworks:**
   Distant patient observing (RPM) frameworks influence remote advances to gather essential sign information from patients in their homes or other non-clinical settings. These frameworks are especially important for people with

persistent circumstances, postoperative patients, or those requiring progressing wellbeing the executives. RPM frameworks normally incorporate wearable gadgets, locally situated sensors, and availability stages that communicate information to medical services suppliers continuously.

For patients with conditions like hypertension or diabetes, RPM permits medical care experts to screen fundamental signs, for example, circulatory strain and glucose levels from a distance. This persistent oversight empowers early location of irregularities, ideal intercession, and acclimations to treatment plans. RPM upgrades patient results as well as diminishes the weight on medical care offices by limiting the requirement for regular in-person visits.

3. **High level Sensors and Biometric Innovations:**

Progressions in sensor advancements have prompted the improvement of additional modern and exact gadgets for essential sign observing. For example, painless ceaseless glucose checking (CGM) gadgets utilize little sensors embedded under the skin to quantify glucose levels over the course of the day. These gadgets offer a huge improvement over customary techniques that require regular fingerstick tests.

Biometric innovations, like facial acknowledgment and infrared sensors, are being incorporated into checking frameworks for painless evaluation of crucial signs. These innovations can quantify boundaries like respiratory rate, pulse, and internal heat level without direct contact, giving a more agreeable and clean insight for people, particularly in high-risk conditions like medical clinics.

4. **Man-made consciousness and Prescient Examination:**

The incorporation of man-made brainpower and AI calculations has improved the investigation of indispensable sign information, empowering more exact expectations and customized medical care experiences. Artificial intelligence driven calculations can handle immense measures of information from ceaseless observing gadgets, distinguish designs, and produce significant experiences.

Prescient examination, specifically, permits medical services experts to expect potential medical problems in view of changes in fundamental signs and other important boundaries.

For instance, AI models can dissect designs in pulse, respiratory rate, and action levels to foresee the probability of a heart occasion or respiratory misery. These prescient capacities are important for people with constant circumstances, considering early mediations and preventive measures. The ceaseless learning nature of man-made intelligence additionally empowers these models to adjust and work on over the long haul as additional information opens up.

5. **Integrative Wellbeing Stages and Electronic Wellbeing Records (EHRs):**

The combination of essential sign observing into extensive wellbeing stages and electronic wellbeing records (EHRs) encourages a more durable and patient-focused way to deal with medical care. Present day wellbeing stages unite information from different sources, including wearables, locally situated sensors, and customary clinical estimations, giving an all encompassing perspective on a singular's wellbeing. This coordinated methodology upholds more educated decision-production by medical services experts.

By connecting crucial sign information straightforwardly to EHRs, medical services suppliers can get to an exhaustive patient history, working with more customized and proficient consideration. For example, a person's verifiable pulse patterns, joined with ongoing movement levels and prescription adherence information, give a nuanced comprehension of their cardiovascular wellbeing. This coordinated methodology smoothes out correspondence between medical care experts and guarantees that fundamental sign information is important for the more extensive patient wellbeing record.

6. **Telehealth and Virtual Consideration:**
   Headways in imperative sign observing have synergized with the development of telehealth and virtual consideration. The capacity to remotely screen fundamental signs and send information continuously upgrades the adequacy of virtual counsels. Telehealth stages frequently coordinate with wearable gadgets and sensors, permitting medical services suppliers to notice changes in fundamental signs during video conferences.

   In remote or underserved regions, telehealth, joined with fundamental sign checking, grows admittance to medical care administrations. People can take part in virtual counsels with medical care experts, share fundamental sign information, and get direction on dealing with their wellbeing. This further develops admittance to mind as well as enables people to partake in their wellbeing the board, cultivating a cooperative methodology among patients and medical services suppliers effectively.

7. **Patient Strengthening and Wellbeing Education:**
   The openness of consistent indispensable sign observing adds to patient strengthening and wellbeing education. People gain a superior comprehension of how their everyday exercises, way of life decisions, and drugs influence their important bodily functions. Wearables and checking frameworks frequently give significant bits of knowledge and wellbeing suggestions, advancing better ways of behaving and way of life adjustments.

   Instructive parts inside checking frameworks can improve wellbeing proficiency by making sense of the meaning of crucial signs and their job in generally speaking prosperity. This expanded mindfulness engages people to settle on informed conclusions about their wellbeing, encouraging a proactive way to deal with preventive consideration and self-administration of constant circumstances.

8. **Administrative Contemplations and Guidelines:**
   The quick advancement of imperative sign observing innovations raises administrative contemplations and the requirement for normalized rehearses. Administrative bodies should adjust to the powerful scene, guaranteeing that these innovations meet rigid security and adequacy principles. The advancement of

clear rules, industry guidelines, and administrative systems is fundamental for encourage development while focusing on understanding security and information protection.

Clinical gadget guideline assumes a pivotal part in guaranteeing the unwavering quality and precision of essential sign checking gadgets. Laying out worldwide guidelines for interoperability and information security is similarly significant, taking into account the worldwide idea of medical services and the potential for cross-line information trade.

9. **Moral Ramifications and Informed Assent:**

The moral ramifications of nonstop imperative sign observing include contemplations connected with security, information possession, and informed assent. People should have a reasonable comprehension of how their important bodily function information will be gathered, put away, and shared. Straightforward and easy to understand assent instruments, combined with hearty information insurance rehearses, are fundamental for address moral worries and construct trust between clients, medical services suppliers, and innovation engineers.

10. **Mix with General Wellbeing Drives:**

Important bodily function checking headways can possibly contribute altogether to general wellbeing drives, particularly with regards to early illness identification and flare-up reconnaissance. Wearables and checking frameworks can act as early advance notice frameworks by recognizing oddities in imperative signs at the populace level. Coordinating crucial sign information into general wellbeing data sets and reconnaissance frameworks can work with a more proactive and information driven reaction to arising wellbeing challenges.

**8.1 In-depth analysis of innovations in vital sign monitoring technologies**

Lately, developments in crucial sign observing advancements have essentially changed the scene of medical care. The combination of cutting edge sensors, wearables, man-made consciousness (artificial intelligence), and network has introduced another period of nonstop and customized wellbeing checking. This top to bottom examination dives into the critical developments in crucial sign observing advancements, investigating their effect on persistent consideration, clinical direction, and the more extensive medical care environment.

1. **Wearables and Constant Observing:**

The coming of wearable gadgets has upset how crucial signs are checked, giving people the capacity to follow their wellbeing continuously. Wearables, for example, smartwatches and wellness trackers, are outfitted with sensors that action boundaries like pulse, blood oxygen levels, and actual work. Consistent checking considers a unique comprehension of imperative signs, moving past disengaged estimations taken during facility visits.

Wearable gadgets have become essential in advancing proactive wellbeing the executives. People can screen their pulse fluctuation, a vital sign of feelings of anxiety and in general cardiovascular wellbeing, over the course of the day. Wearables with rest following capacities offer bits of knowledge into rest quality, assisting clients with understanding the effect of their rest designs on by and large prosperity. These persistent checking capacities engage people to go with informed way of life decisions and identify early indications of potential medical problems.

2. **Distant Patient Checking (RPM) Frameworks:**
   Distant Patient Checking (RPM) frameworks influence availability and wearable sensors to empower medical care suppliers to screen patients' important bodily functions from a distance. This advancement is especially important for people with ongoing circumstances or those recuperating from medical procedures, considering nonstop oversight without the requirement for continuous clinic visits. RPM frameworks commonly incorporate wearable gadgets, locally established sensors, and secure information transmission to medical services suppliers.

   RPM upgrades patient consideration by working with early recognition of peculiarities and opportune mediations. For example, patients with hypertension can have their circulatory strain observed consistently without leaving their homes. This persistent information stream empowers medical care suppliers to change prescription regimens, offer virtual conferences, and give customized care plans. RPM works on persistent results as well as decreases the burden on medical care assets, limiting the requirement for clinic affirmations.

3. **High level Sensor Advancements:**
   Developments in sensor advances have made ready for more precise and refined crucial sign checking. Consistent Glucose Observing (CGM) gadgets, for instance, use little sensors embedded under the skin to quantify glucose levels over the course of the day. This approach replaces conventional fingerstick tests, offering a more helpful and persistent checking answer for people with diabetes. Biometric sensors, for example, those coordinated into savvy attire or fixes, give harmless checking of indispensable signs. These sensors can gauge boundaries like respiratory rate, pulse, and internal heat level without the requirement for direct skin contact. This development is especially significant in situations where solace and cleanliness are fundamental, like in clinic settings or for long haul wear.

4. **Computerized reasoning (simulated intelligence) and Prescient Examination:**
   The joining of simulated intelligence and AI in crucial sign checking has introduced another time of information examination and understanding. Simulated intelligence calculations can handle huge datasets created by ceaseless observing gadgets, distinguish designs, and give prescient bits of knowledge into an

individual's wellbeing. Prescient examination, fueled by artificial intelligence, considers the expectation of potential medical problems in view of changes in fundamental signs and other significant boundaries.

For instance, AI models can examine designs in pulse, respiratory rate, and actual work to anticipate the beginning of a cardiovascular occasion or respiratory pain. These prescient capacities empower medical services suppliers to intercede proactively, forestalling unfavorable results and working on understanding consideration. The ceaseless learning nature of artificial intelligence calculations likewise guarantees that forecasts become more refined and precise over the long haul as additional information opens up.

5. **Joining with Electronic Wellbeing Records (EHRs):**

The consistent joining of crucial sign checking information into Electronic Wellbeing Records (EHRs) is an essential headway that improves the congruity of care. Present day wellbeing stages unite information from different sources, including wearables, locally established sensors, and conventional clinical estimations. This reconciliation guarantees that medical services suppliers approach an exhaustive patient history, encouraging more educated direction.

Connecting indispensable sign information straightforwardly to EHRs gives an all encompassing perspective on a patient's wellbeing. For instance, a doctor can survey verifiable pulse patterns, late active work levels, and prescription adherence information in a bound together connection point.

This coordinated methodology smoothes out correspondence between medical services experts, lessens the gamble of information storehouses, and guarantees that fundamental sign information is a necessary piece of the patient's more extensive wellbeing record.

6. **Telehealth and Virtual Consideration Reconciliation:**

The development of imperative sign checking innovations has synergized with the development of telehealth and virtual consideration. The capacity to remotely screen crucial signs and communicate information progressively upgrades the adequacy of virtual discussions. Telehealth stages frequently coordinate with wearable gadgets and sensors, permitting medical care suppliers to notice changes in imperative signs during video discussions.

In situations where in-person visits are testing, for example, during a worldwide pandemic, virtual consideration turns into a basic part of medical services conveyance. The coordination of crucial sign observing with telehealth guarantees that medical services suppliers can survey patients from a distance, settle on information informed choices, and give opportune intercessions. This joining further develops admittance to mind as well as upgrades the general effectiveness of medical care conveyance.

7. **Patient Strengthening through Information Access:**

One of the significant effects of imperative sign checking developments is the strengthening of patients through direct admittance to their wellbeing information. Wearable gadgets and observing frameworks frequently accompany easy to use connection points and versatile applications that give people ongoing bits of knowledge into their important bodily functions. This democratization of wellbeing information encourages a feeling of pride and responsibility for one's prosperity.

Patients can effectively take part in their wellbeing the board by putting forth private wellbeing objectives, following advancement, and getting customized suggestions in view of their important bodily function information. The openness of this data upgrades wellbeing proficiency, empowering people to come to informed conclusions about their ways of life, medicine adherence, and generally speaking wellbeing. This shift towards patient-focused care lines up with a more extensive pattern in medical services that underlines coordinated effort among patients and medical care suppliers.

8. **Administrative Contemplations and Principles:**
   The quick advancement of imperative sign observing innovations requires clear administrative systems and norms to guarantee wellbeing, viability, and moral use. Clinical gadget guideline assumes an essential part in approving the precision and unwavering quality of these innovations. Administrative bodies should adjust to the powerful scene, adjusting the requirement for advancement with the basic to safeguard patient security and information protection.

   Laying out global norms for interoperability, information security, and moral contemplations is significant for encouraging a firm environment. The improvement of rules that incorporate the different scope of imperative sign checking innovations, from wearables to cutting edge sensors, gives a guide to producers, medical care suppliers, and controllers. Consistence with these principles guarantees that developments in imperative sign checking are lined up with the most elevated levels of value and patient consideration.

9. **Moral Ramifications and Informed Assent:**
   The moral contemplations related with crucial sign observing innovations include issues of protection, information proprietorship, and informed assent. People should have a reasonable comprehension of how their important bodily function information will be gathered, put away, and shared. Straightforward and easy to use assent instruments, combined with powerful information assurance rehearses, are crucial for address moral worries and fabricate trust between clients, medical care suppliers, and innovation designers.

   Moral contemplations likewise reach out to issues of value and availability. Guaranteeing that fundamental sign observing advances are available to different populaces, incorporating those with changing financial status or innovative proficiency, is essential to forestall the compounding of existing medical care incongruities. Moral systems should direct the turn of events and organization of these innovations to guarantee that they contribute emphatically to medical services results for all people.

## 10. Future Bearings and Difficulties:

As developments in essential sign observing advancements keep on unfurling, a few future bearings and provokes come to the very front. The reconciliation of numerous information streams, for example, genomics, way of life factors, and ecological information, holds the potential for a more all encompassing comprehension of wellbeing. The test lies in creating thorough models that can examine and decipher this complex information in a significant and noteworthy manner.

Interoperability stays a constant test, especially as the environment of imperative sign observing gadgets keeps on enhancing. Normalizing information designs, correspondence conventions, and gadget connection points is critical for guaranteeing consistent joining into more extensive medical services frameworks. Cooperative endeavors between industry partners, innovation engineers, and administrative bodies are fundamental for address these interoperability challenges.

The moral ramifications of prescient examination and computer based intelligence driven experiences likewise warrant continuous thought. Finding some kind of harmony between utilizing these advancements for proactive medical care mediations and regarding individual independence is a developing test. Guaranteeing that people have organization over their wellbeing information and that the utilization of prescient investigation lines up with moral standards is basic for the dependable arrangement of these advancements.

### 8.2 Exploration of non-invasive and continuous monitoring devices

The investigation of harmless and constant checking gadgets addresses a historic boondocks in medical care, offering a change in outlook from customary irregular estimations to ongoing, nonstop bits of knowledge into fundamental signs and wellbeing boundaries. These creative gadgets influence progressed sensor advances, wearables, and network to give an abundance of information, engaging both medical care experts and people to screen wellbeing in a more complete and proactive way. This inside and out investigation analyzes the importance, applications, and ramifications of painless and consistent observing gadgets across different medical services spaces.

1. **Meaning of Harmless Ceaseless Checking:**
   Harmless ceaseless checking gadgets hold critical significance in present day medical services because of their capacity to give a constant stream of continuous information without the requirement for obtrusive methods. Conventional strategies frequently include discontinuous estimations, for example, intermittent pulse readings or incidental electrocardiograms. Conversely, painless persistent checking empowers a more unique and all encompassing comprehension of a singular's wellbeing by catching continuous varieties in essential signs and physiological boundaries.

   The meaning of these gadgets is especially apparent with regards to persistent sicknesses, where nonstop checking considers early identification of irregularities and opportune mediations. For example, people with hypertension can profit from constant circulatory strain checking, empowering medical services experts to recognize patterns, change drugs, and give customized care plans. The persistent idea of checking likewise works with a more nuanced evaluation of wellbeing, taking into account factors like circadian rhythms, stress reactions, and changes in action levels.

2. **Applications in Cardiovascular Wellbeing:**
   Harmless constant observing gadgets assume an essential part in cardiovascular wellbeing, offering experiences into boundaries, for example, pulse, circulatory strain, and cadence. Wearable gadgets furnished with photoplethysmography (PPG) sensors empower persistent checking of pulse by estimating changes in blood volume under the skin.

   This innovation gives a more exhaustive perspective on pulse elements over the course of the day, uncovering designs that might slip through the cracks in irregular estimations.

   For people with arrhythmias or those in danger of cardiovascular occasions, persistent electrocardiogram (ECG or EKG) it are instrumental to screen gadgets. These gadgets can recognize anomalies in heart cadence, empowering early mediation and avoidance of possibly hazardous occasions. The information gathered by consistent checking gadgets in cardiovascular wellbeing helps with clinical navigation as well as engages people to effectively deal with their heart wellbeing by making way of life changes and sticking to treatment plans.

3. **Constant Glucose Observing in Diabetes The executives:**
   Harmless constant checking has altered diabetes the executives through Ceaseless Glucose Observing (CGM) gadgets. Customarily, people with diabetes depended on irregular fingerstick tests to gauge blood glucose levels. CGM gadgets, then again, utilize little sensors embedded under the skin to persistently screen glucose levels over the course of the day. This approach gives a more exact and nuanced image of glucose elements, assisting people with coming to informed conclusions about insulin measurements, dietary decisions, and by and large diabetes self-administration.

   The nonstop idea of glucose observing is especially gainful for people with fluctuating glucose levels, like those with Type 1 diabetes. It empowers the recognition of patterns and examples, prompting convenient changes in insulin treatment. Furthermore, CGM gadgets can make people aware of potential hypoglycemic or hyperglycemic episodes, lessening the gamble of serious inconveniences. The incorporation of CGM information into computerized wellbeing stages further improves correspondence between people with diabetes and their medical services suppliers.

4. **Respiratory Checking for Respiratory Circumstances:**
   Harmless constant observing stretches out its applications to respiratory well-

being, giving important experiences into boundaries like respiratory rate, oxygen immersion, and breathing examples. Wearable gadgets with worked in accelerometers and respiratory sensors can identify changes in respiratory examples, making them helpful for people with respiratory circumstances like ongoing obstructive aspiratory illness (COPD) or asthma.

Persistent heartbeat oximetry, which estimates oxygen immersion levels, is significant for checking people with respiratory split the difference. Wearable heartbeat oximeters can give continuous information on oxygen levels, supporting the early recognition of respiratory trouble. For patients recuperating from medical procedures or overseeing persistent respiratory circumstances, constant checking gadgets offer a proactive way to deal with medical services, considering opportune intercessions and diminishing the gamble of intensifications.

5. **Rest Checking and Rest Problems:**
   Harmless ceaseless observing gadgets have found applications in the domain of rest wellbeing, offering bits of knowledge into rest examples, quality, and potential rest problems. Wearable gadgets outfitted with accelerometers and photoplethysmography sensors can screen developments, pulse, and oxygen immersion levels during rest. This information is instrumental in evaluating rest design and distinguishing aggravations like rest apnea or a propensity to fidget.

   Persistent rest observing adds to the conclusion and the executives of rest problems by giving a far reaching perspective on a singular's rest propensities. The information can be utilized to identify examples of a sleeping disorder, survey the viability of rest mediations, and guide customized suggestions for further developing rest cleanliness. People can acquire a superior comprehension of their rest quality, working with way of life changes for improved generally prosperity.

6. **Maternal and Fetal Checking in Obstetrics:**
   In obstetrics, painless consistent checking gadgets assume a critical part in maternal and fetal wellbeing. Wearable gadgets and particular sensors empower consistent checking of maternal indispensable signs, uterine withdrawals, and fetal pulse. This approach upgrades the early discovery of possible complexities during pregnancy and work, considering opportune intercessions to guarantee the prosperity of both the mother and the child.

   Persistent fetal pulse checking, for example, gives significant bits of knowledge into the child's cardiovascular wellbeing and reaction to withdrawals during work. Wearable gadgets furnished with uterine action sensors add to the appraisal of work movement. These checking advancements upgrade the wellbeing and accuracy of obstetric consideration, enabling medical care experts to settle on informed choices and giving eager guardians consolation.

7. **Difficulties and Contemplations in Harmless Ceaseless Observing:**
   While harmless ceaseless observing gadgets offer momentous headways, they are not without difficulties and contemplations. Protection and information

security are principal concerns, particularly as these gadgets gather delicate well-being data. Guaranteeing strong encryption, secure information stockpiling, and rigid access controls are basic to safeguard people's protection and conform to medical care guidelines.

Another test is the requirement for normalization and interoperability among different observing gadgets. Various producers might utilize exclusive innovations, making it trying to incorporate information from different sources into a strong wellbeing record. Laying out industry norms and advancing interoperability are fundamental stages in making a consistent environment where information from various gadgets can be totaled and broke down extensively.

Besides, tending to the moral ramifications of constant checking, like informed assent and client independence, is basic. People should be very much informed about how their wellbeing information will be utilized, and they ought to can handle the sharing of their data. Finding some kind of harmony between utilizing the advantages of persistent checking and regarding individual independence is fundamental for building trust in these advancements.

## 8. Future Headings and Combination with Advanced Wellbeing Stages:

The eventual fate of harmless consistent checking is ready for additional development and reconciliation with advanced wellbeing stages. As innovation progresses, these checking gadgets are probably going to turn out to be more refined, offering extra boundaries and experiences. Coordination with man-made brainpower (simulated intelligence) calculations will upgrade the capacity to examine complex datasets, giving more precise expectations and customized wellbeing suggestions.

The combination of ceaseless observing information into computerized wellbeing stages and Electronic Wellbeing Records (EHRs) will work with a more all encompassing way to deal with medical services. Medical services experts will approach far reaching datasets that length imperative signs, way of life factors, and genomic data, empowering a more customized and exact way to deal with conclusion and therapy. This joining likewise enables people to effectively participate in their wellbeing the board, going with informed choices in light of a comprehensive comprehension of their prosperity.

### 8.3 Discussion on the role of wearables, sensors, and other technologies in advancing vital sign monitoring

The job of wearables, sensors, and different advancements in progressing fundamental sign observing is groundbreaking, introducing a time of customized, persistent medical services. These advancements influence state of the art innovations to give constant information on key physiological boundaries, engaging the two people and medical care experts with phenomenal experiences into wellbeing and prosperity. This conversation investigates the multi-layered effect of wearables, sensors, and related advancements in progressing imperative sign observing across different medical services areas.

1. **Wearables Altering Individual Wellbeing Observing:**
Wearables, for example, smartwatches and wellness trackers, have become pervasive in the public eye, with their job reaching out past simple assistants to strong wellbeing observing apparatuses.
Outfitted with sensors like accelerometers, gyrators, and pulse screens, wearables give ceaseless information on actual work, rest designs, and important bodily functions. This ongoing criticism empowers people to adopt a proactive strategy to their wellbeing, cultivating a culture of mindfulness and prosperity.
Pulse checking, a standard component in numerous wearables, offers bits of knowledge into cardiovascular wellbeing. Clients can follow resting pulse, work out actuated pulse changeability, and even distinguish anomalies in heart musicality. Such persistent checking is instrumental in distinguishing patterns, provoking way of life changes, and working with early mediations for likely cardiovascular issues. Wearables in this way engage people to deal with their heart wellbeing consistently effectively.

2. **Sensors Empowering Constant Physiological Observing:**
The combination of cutting edge sensors assumes a crucial part in extending the extent of essential sign observing past conventional boundaries. Photoplethysmography (PPG) sensors, for instance, utilize light to gauge blood volume changes under the skin, giving ceaseless pulse checking without the requirement for chest lashes or terminals. These sensors are regularly tracked down in wearables and are progressively coordinated into different wellbeing checking gadgets.
Notwithstanding pulse, sensors can screen other imperative signs, for example, blood oxygen levels and skin temperature. Wearables with SpO2 sensors offer nonstop oxygen immersion observing, especially applicable for people with respiratory circumstances or those adapting to high elevations. Skin temperature observing gives experiences into circadian rhythms and can be used to distinguish fever or varieties related with hormonal changes.

3. **Nonstop Glucose Observing Changing Diabetes Care:**
Ceaseless Glucose Checking (CGM) represents the groundbreaking effect of sensor innovation in diabetes the executives. CGM gadgets use small sensors embedded under the skin to gauge glucose levels over the course of the day, giving a nonstop stream of information. This development replaces conventional fingerstick tests, offering a more exhaustive comprehension of glucose elements and limiting the requirement for regular intrusive estimations.
The constant information from CGM gadgets empowers people with diabetes to arrive at informed conclusions about insulin measurements, dietary decisions, and way of life adjustments. Medical care experts can remotely screen

glucose patterns, mediate proactively, and change therapy plans. CGM gadgets represent how ceaseless observing, empowered by sensor innovation, works on the accuracy of diabetes the executives and upgrades the personal satisfaction for people with the condition.

4. **Man-made reasoning Upgrading Information Examination:**

   The coordination of man-made reasoning (artificial intelligence) calculations improves the investigation of tremendous datasets created by wearables and sensors, separating significant experiences and forecasts. Man-made intelligence driven investigation can recognize examples, inconsistencies, and connections inside ceaseless checking information, offering a degree of refinement that customary techniques can't coordinate. This ability is especially important in foreseeing wellbeing results, empowering customized mediations, and enhancing medical services conveyance.

   For example, man-made intelligence calculations can examine pulse fluctuation information to anticipate the gamble of cardiovascular occasions or survey feelings of anxiety. AI models can identify unpretentious changes in crucial signs that might go before medical problems, considering early mediation and preventive measures. The persistent learning nature of man-made intelligence guarantees that these models advance after some time, adjusting to individual wellbeing directions and refining their prescient abilities.

5. **Far off Persistent Checking Upgrading Medical services Openness:**

   The collaboration of wearables, sensors, and availability advances adds to the development of Far off Quiet Observing (RPM) frameworks. These frameworks empower medical services suppliers to screen patients' important bodily functions and wellbeing measurements, encouraging a more proactive and patient-focused way to deal with care from a distance. Wearables furnished with RPM capacities, related to get information transmission, make a consistent association among people and their medical services groups.

   RPM is especially significant for overseeing ongoing circumstances, postoperative consideration, and observing high-risk populaces. Patients can approach their regular routines while their important bodily functions are ceaselessly communicated to medical care suppliers. This not just decreases the requirement for successive in-person visits yet additionally works with early recognition of oddities, empowering convenient mediations and forestalling hospitalizations. RPM epitomizes how innovation driven nonstop observing broadens medical services past conventional clinical settings.

6. **Wearables in Emotional well-being Checking:**

   Past actual wellbeing, wearables and sensors are progressively assuming a part in checking mental prosperity. High level sensors, including those estimating skin conductance, internal heat level, and development designs, can give marks of feelings of anxiety, nervousness, and rest quality. Wearables outfitted with these sensors offer a non-nosy method for persistently observing psychological wellness boundaries.

Nonstop observing of psychological well-being considers a more comprehensive comprehension of a singular's general prosperity. For instance, changes in rest designs or expanded feelings of anxiety distinguished by wearables can provoke early mediations or way of life changes. Coordinating psychological wellness boundaries into the continuum of nonstop observing mirrors the advancing scene of customized and far reaching medical care.

7. **Difficulties and Contemplations in Persistent Observing Advancements:**
   While the headways in wearables, sensors, and persistent observing advancements are promising, a few difficulties and contemplations merit consideration. Security concerns connected with the assortment and capacity of delicate well-being information stay a noticeable issue. Guaranteeing vigorous encryption, secure information transmission, and adherence to severe protection guidelines are basic to assemble and keep up with trust among clients.

   Interoperability is another test, particularly as the biological system of checking gadgets differentiates. Normalizing information designs, correspondence conventions, and gadget points of interaction is critical for consistent combination into more extensive medical services frameworks. Joint effort among producers, medical care suppliers, and administrative bodies is fundamental to lay out industry norms that work with the trading of data across different stages.

   Moral contemplations, including informed assent, client independence, and capable information use, should be at the bleeding edge of nonstop observing innovations. People ought to have clear data about how their information will be used, and they ought to hold command over the sharing of their data. Finding some kind of harmony between the advantages of nonstop checking and regarding individual protection and independence is basic for the moral organization of these advancements.

8. **Future Headings and Coordination with Environments:**

The fate of ceaseless observing advancements holds invigorating possibilities, with continuous developments and mix into more extensive wellbeing biological systems. Wearables and sensors are probably going to turn out to be more complex, offering a more extensive cluster of boundaries for checking. The mix of ceaseless observing information with Electronic Wellbeing Records (EHRs) and other computerized wellbeing stages will empower a more far reaching and strong way to deal with medical services.

As the field progresses, the improvement of novel sensors for observing extra wellbeing boundaries, for example, hydration levels, electrolyte balance, or ecological openings, is expected. Wearables might advance to integrate increased reality (AR) or computer generated reality (VR) highlights, giving vivid wellbeing encounters and upgrading client commitment. The potential for wearables and constant observing advances to flawlessly coordinate into day to day existence, giving significant bits of knowledge and customized proposals, positions them as foundation components in store for medical services.

**8.4 Implications for preventive healthcare and early disease detection**

The ramifications of persistent checking innovations for preventive medical care and early infection recognition are significant, proclaiming a change in outlook from receptive to proactive medical services models. These innovations, enveloping wearables, sensors, and high level information examination, engage people and medical care experts with ongoing bits of knowledge into wellbeing boundaries. This conversation investigates the extraordinary effect of constant observing on preventive medical services and early infection recognition, stressing the possibility to move the medical care center from overseeing sicknesses to forestalling them.

1. **Proactive Wellbeing The executives Through Ceaseless Observing:**

   Nonstop observing advancements establish the groundwork for proactive wellbeing the board by giving people the apparatuses to effectively take part in their prosperity. Wearables, furnished with sensors that track essential signs, active work, and rest designs, empower clients to acquire an extensive comprehension of their wellbeing on an everyday premise. This proactive methodology cultivates a culture of counteraction, empowering people to go with informed way of life decisions and intercessions before medical problems raise.

   For example, constant observing of pulse inconstancy can offer experiences into feelings of anxiety and in general cardiovascular wellbeing. Furnished with this data, people can execute pressure the board methods, alter their work-out schedules, or change their rest propensities to address potential gamble factors. The capacity to distinguish unobtrusive changes in wellbeing boundaries engages people to go to preventive lengths, diminishing the probability of creating persistent circumstances and advancing generally prosperity.

2. **Early Identification of Abnormalities and Infection Forerunners:**

   Persistent checking innovations act as watchful sentinels, continually noticing wellbeing boundaries for irregularities and early indications of potential medical problems. The reconciliation of sensors that screen pulse, circulatory strain, glucose levels, and other crucial signs takes into account the early discovery of deviations from standard qualities. This early discovery is especially critical in distinguishing illness antecedents and starting mediations before side effects manifest.

   With regards to cardiovascular wellbeing, consistent checking can identify anomalies in heart cadence that might go before a heart occasion. Early intercession in view of such cautions can forestall serious results and work on understanding results. Also, constant glucose observing works with the early ID of changes in glucose levels, empowering people and medical care suppliers to make convenient acclimations to diabetes the board plans.

3. **Ongoing Infection The board and Counteraction:**
   Persistent checking innovations assume a crucial part in the administration and counteraction of constant illnesses. For people with conditions like diabetes, hypertension, or respiratory issues, constant checking gives a dynamic and ongoing comprehension of wellbeing boundaries. This empowers customized infection the board plans, taking into account the ideal change of drugs, way of life adjustments, and proactive mediations to forestall sickness movement.

   The proactive administration of constant circumstances adds to better wellbeing results and a more excellent of life. People can effectively take part in their consideration by sticking to treatment plans, pursuing informed choices in light of constant checking information, and teaming up with medical services experts in a common dynamic model. Counteraction techniques, informed by constant checking bits of knowledge, become vital in alleviating the drawn out effect of persistent sicknesses.

4. **Accuracy in Customized Medication:**
   Persistent checking innovations add to the worldview of customized medication by giving exact, individualized bits of knowledge into wellbeing boundaries. The granularity of information created by wearables and sensors empowers medical care experts to tailor mediations in light of a singular's special wellbeing profile. This accuracy considers designated preventive measures and early recognition methodologies that line up with the particular requirements and attributes of every individual.

   For instance, people with differing reactions to stress might profit from customized pressure the executives intercessions in light of ceaseless checking of pulse fluctuation. Accuracy in diabetes the executives can include changing insulin doses in view of continuous glucose patterns, improving glycemic control. The capacity to fit preventive systems to individual wellbeing profiles upgrades the viability of medical services mediations and adds to the general outcome of preventive medical care endeavors.

5. **Information Driven Bits of knowledge for Medical care Suppliers:**
   Consistent checking innovations enable people as well as furnish medical care suppliers with an abundance of information driven experiences. The mix of consistent observing information into Electronic Wellbeing Records (EHRs) and wellbeing data frameworks upgrades the capacity of medical care experts to pursue informed clinical choices. Continuous information on indispensable signs, patterns, and oddities work with an exhaustive comprehension of a patient's wellbeing status.

   Medical services suppliers can use these bits of knowledge for early infection recognition, preventive consideration arranging, and convenient mediations. For example, oddities in constant glucose observing information can provoke changes in accordance with diabetes the board plans during virtual conferences.

Distant Patient Observing (RPM) frameworks, empowered by consistent checking advances, expand the scope of medical care administrations, particularly for people with constant circumstances or those in far off areas.

6. **General Wellbeing Drives and Populace Wellbeing The executives:**
Nonstop checking advancements have more extensive ramifications for general wellbeing drives and populace wellbeing the executives. Collected and anonymized information from wearables and sensors can add to the observation of populace wellbeing patterns. This information can be utilized to distinguish arising medical problems, evaluate the viability of preventive measures, and designer general wellbeing mediations in view of constant bits of knowledge.

For instance, patterns in pulse changeability or respiratory examples from a populace can give early signs of feelings of anxiety or respiratory circumstances. General wellbeing specialists can utilize this data to send designated mediations, dispense assets proficiently, and execute preventive measures at a populace level. The incorporation of constant checking information into populace wellbeing the executives systems improves the deftness and responsiveness of general wellbeing drives.

7. **Difficulties and Contemplations in Preventive Medical care with Nonstop Observing:**

While the likely advantages of nonstop checking innovations for preventive medical services are critical, difficulties and contemplations should be tended to. Protection concerns, information security, and the mindful utilization of wellbeing information are vital. Carrying out powerful encryption, secure information transmission, and clear information administration systems are crucial for construct and keep up with trust among people and guarantee the moral sending of these innovations.

Another thought is the advanced separation, as not all people have equivalent admittance to or capability in utilizing persistent checking advances. Tending to variations in innovation access, computerized proficiency, and medical services education is vital to guarantee that the advantages of persistent checking stretch out to assorted populaces. Furthermore, the requirement for administrative structures, interoperability norms, and moral rules stays vital to the mindful combination of nonstop checking innovations into medical services frameworks.

# Chapter 9

## The Future of Wellness Tech

The fate of health tech guarantees a groundbreaking excursion, mixing state of the art innovations with an all encompassing way to deal with individual prosperity. From cutting edge wearables and customized nourishment to vivid encounters and man-made consciousness (computer based intelligence) coordination, the scene of health innovation is advancing quickly. This investigation dives into the multi-layered features representing things to come of wellbeing tech, featuring key patterns, advancements, and the expected effect on people's wellbeing and way of life.

1. **Comprehensive Wellbeing Environments:**
   The fate of health tech imagines the making of all encompassing biological systems that flawlessly coordinate different advances to address assorted parts of prosperity. These environments go past detached gadgets, shaping interconnected networks that consider physical, mental, and profound wellbeing. High level wearables, brilliant home gadgets, versatile applications, and virtual stages meet to completely make a brought together encounter that takes care of individual necessities.

   For example, a comprehensive wellbeing biological system could consolidate a savvy wearable that screens active work, rest, and feelings of anxiety, close by a sustenance application that gives customized dietary suggestions. These interconnected innovations share information, furnishing clients and medical services experts with a comprehensive perspective on a singular's prosperity. The reconciliation of information across numerous aspects empowers a more nuanced comprehension of wellbeing, encouraging proactive and customized mediations.

2. **High level Wearables and Wellbeing Following:**
   The development of wearables addresses a foundation representing things to come of wellbeing tech. Past straightforward movement trackers, high level wearables are turning out to be more modern, integrating a different scope of

sensors to screen different wellbeing boundaries. These wearables go past counting steps; they measure pulse inconstancy, track rest cycles, and evaluate feelings of anxiety. The joining of persistent observing innovations gives constant experiences, enabling people to deal with their wellbeing on an everyday premise effectively.

Future wearables are probably going to include upgraded biometric sensors for more exact wellbeing following. For example, wearables with harmless blood glucose checking abilities could alter diabetes the executives. The consistent joining of wearables into day to day existence urges a proactive way to deal with wellbeing, with people getting significant experiences that empower them to pursue informed choices in regards to their way of life, exercise, and stress the executives.

3. **Customized Sustenance and Wellbeing Plans:**

The fate of health tech embraces the idea of customized nourishment, perceiving that singular prosperity is impacted by interesting dietary necessities. Trend setting innovations, including computer based intelligence and AI, investigate factors like hereditary qualities, digestion, and dietary inclinations to make customized sustenance plans. These plans think about the dietary substance as well as the timing and recurrence of feasts, lining up with a person's circadian rhythms and way of life.

The reconciliation of customized sustenance applications with savvy kitchen apparatuses and feast conveyance benefits further smoothes out the most common way of taking on customized dietary proposals. Shrewd coolers can give continuous stock of food things, and associated kitchen gadgets can direct clients through the planning of dinners lined up with their wholesome requirements. The combination of innovation and sustenance holds the possibility to upset dietary propensities, adding to long haul wellbeing and health.

4. **Vivid Wellbeing Encounters:**

The eventual fate of health tech stretches out past actual wellbeing, consolidating vivid encounters to upgrade mental and profound prosperity. Computer generated reality (VR) and expanded reality (AR) innovations assume a critical part in making vivid wellbeing encounters. VR reflection applications, for instance, transport clients to peaceful conditions, cultivating unwinding and stress decrease. AR applications can overlay genuine conditions with data and signs to help careful living.

These vivid encounters stretch out to wellness too, with VR-based exercises giving drawing in and dynamic work-out schedules. The gamification of wellness encounters through VR makes practice more agreeable as well as urges consistency and adherence to health schedules. The combination of vivid innovations into health methodologies mirrors an all encompassing comprehension of wellbeing, perceiving the interconnectedness of physical and mental prosperity.

5. **Man-made reasoning for Customized Wellbeing Experiences:**

Computerized reasoning is ready to be a main thrust in store for wellbeing tech, giving customized wellbeing bits of knowledge and prescient examination. Simulated intelligence calculations dissect tremendous datasets from wearables, wellbeing trackers, and other checking gadgets to recognize examples, connections, and potential wellbeing gambles. This investigation goes past basic information following, offering people and medical services experts significant experiences into wellbeing patterns and customized proposals.

For example, simulated intelligence driven calculations can anticipate potential medical problems in view of changes in rest designs, movement levels, and physiological boundaries. The coordination of man-made intelligence with electronic wellbeing records (EHRs) further upgrades the capacity of medical services suppliers to offer customized care plans. The ceaseless learning nature of simulated intelligence guarantees that proposals develop with individual wellbeing directions, adding to proactive wellbeing the board.

6. **Psychological wellness Tech and Stress The executives:**
   The eventual fate of wellbeing tech puts a critical accentuation on psychological wellness, perceiving the multifaceted association between mental prosperity and in general wellbeing. Psychological well-being tech arrangements, including care applications, stress trackers, and temperament observing apparatuses, are becoming necessary parts of health environments. Wearables with biosensors can recognize physiological markers of stress, provoking ideal mediations, for example, directed reflection meetings or unwinding works out.

   Man-made intelligence fueled emotional well-being chatbots and virtual specialists offer available and customized help. These advances influence normal language handling and AI to comprehend and answer clients' personal states. The combination of emotional wellness tech into day to day existence empowers a proactive and destigmatized way to deal with mental prosperity, cultivating a culture where people effectively focus on and deal with their psychological well-being.

7. **Blockchain for Wellbeing Information Security:**
   As wellbeing tech depends progressively on the assortment and examination of touchy wellbeing information, guaranteeing the security and protection of this data is central.

   Blockchain innovation arises as a likely arrangement, giving a decentralized and secure structure for overseeing wellbeing information. Blockchain permits people to have more noteworthy command over their wellbeing data, conceding authorization for explicit substances to access and utilize their information while keeping up with protection and security.

   Blockchain's alter safe nature upgrades the uprightness of wellbeing records, forestalling unapproved changes. This decentralized methodology lines up with the standards of client driven command over private information, relieving concerns connected with information breaks and unapproved access. Coordinating blockchain into wellbeing tech biological systems adds to building trust among clients, encouraging a solid and straightforward climate for wellbeing information the executives.

8. **Biofeedback and Neurotechnology:**
   Biofeedback and neurotechnology are arising as key parts representing things to come of health tech, offering people bits of knowledge into their physiological and neurological reactions. Wearable gadgets furnished with biofeedback sensors, for example, those estimating pulse inconstancy or skin conductance, give continuous input on feelings of anxiety and profound states. Clients can then participate in mediations, like profound breathing activities or directed contemplation, to tweak their physiological reactions.

   Neurotechnology, including mind detecting wearables and neurofeedback gadgets, permits people to screen and prepare their cerebrum movement. These advancements have applications in pressure decrease, mental improvement, and rest enhancement. The joining of biofeedback and neurotechnology into wellbeing biological systems upholds a comprehensive way to deal with wellbeing, empowering people to effectively take part in their prosperity by understanding and directing both physiological and neurological perspectives.

9. **Difficulties and Contemplations coming soon for Wellbeing Tech:**
   While the eventual fate of wellbeing tech holds gigantic commitment, a few difficulties and contemplations should be tended to for far reaching reception and ideal effect. Protection concerns connected with the assortment and utilization of individual wellbeing information require hearty shields. Carrying out straightforward information administration works on, acquiring informed assent, and guaranteeing consistence with protection guidelines are fundamental stages in building and keeping up with client trust.

   Interoperability stays a test as the health tech scene enhances. Coordinating information from different gadgets, stages, and applications into firm wellbeing environments requires normalized information configurations and correspondence conventions. Cooperation among tech engineers, medical services suppliers, and administrative bodies is critical in laying out interoperability norms that work with the consistent trade of data.

   Moral contemplations encompassing computer based intelligence and AI calculations require cautious consideration. Guaranteeing reasonableness, straightforwardness, and responsibility in algorithmic dynamic cycles is basic. Finding some kind of harmony between the advantages of man-made intelligence driven customized bits of knowledge and the moral utilization of information is fundamental for building client certainty and confidence in wellbeing tech arrangements.

10. **Future Wellbeing Tech and Comprehensive Access:**

As the eventual fate of health tech unfurls, guaranteeing comprehensive access for different populaces turns into a basic thought. Tending to differences in innovation access, advanced proficiency, and medical services education is fundamental to forestall the fuel of existing wellbeing disparities. Engineers, policymakers, and medical services suppliers should work cooperatively to plan arrangements that take care of different necessities, taking into account factors like financial status, social foundations, and shifting degrees of innovative capability.

Comprehensive plan standards ought to be at the bleeding edge of creating health tech answers for guarantee availability for people with incapacities. This incorporates contemplations, for example, planning UIs that are traversable for people with visual impedances or guaranteeing similarity with assistive advances.

### 9.1 Overview of emerging trends and technologies in wellness tech

The health tech scene is going through a unique change, driven by an intermingling of arising patterns and innovations that expect to reclassify how people approach and focus on their prosperity. This outline digs into the diverse aspects of the developing wellbeing tech space, investigating key patterns and advances that are forming the business and upsetting the manner in which individuals deal with their wellbeing and way of life.

1. **Customized Health Arrangements:**

   One of the noticeable patterns in wellbeing tech is the shift towards customized arrangements that take care of individual wellbeing needs and inclinations. Propels in information examination, AI, and computerized reasoning engage wellbeing tech stages to dissect tremendous datasets, including biometric data, way of life decisions, and hereditary information. This investigation empowers the making of profoundly customized health plans, covering regions like nourishment, wellness, stress the executives, and rest.

   Customized nourishment applications, for example, use calculations to survey clients' dietary propensities, wholesome prerequisites, and wellbeing objectives to offer redid dinner plans. Additionally, wellness applications influence individual information, including action levels and exercise inclinations, to tailor gym routine schedules.

   This pattern mirrors a developing acknowledgment that one-size-fits-all ways to deal with wellbeing are inadequate, and people are looking for arrangements that line up with their exceptional physiological cosmetics and way of life.

2. **Joining of Wearables and Wellbeing Trackers:**

   Wearable gadgets and wellbeing trackers have become fundamental parts of the wellbeing tech scene, offering clients continuous bits of knowledge into their wellbeing and movement levels. These gadgets, going from smartwatches to wellness trackers, are furnished with a variety of sensors that screen different biometric boundaries, including pulse, rest designs, and actual work. The joining of wearables into day to day existence urges a proactive way to deal with wellbeing, with people getting ceaseless criticism and significant experiences.

High level wearables go past fundamental following, integrating highlights like electrocardiogram (ECG) observing, blood oxygen level estimation, and even pressure following. These capacities give a far reaching perspective on a singular's wellbeing, empowering early recognition of possible issues and working with proactive mediations. As wearables keep on developing, their mix with other health tech stages makes a comprehensive environment that upholds people in dealing with various parts of their prosperity.

3. **Telehealth and Virtual Wellbeing Stages:**

The ascent of telehealth and virtual wellbeing stages has been advanced by innovative progressions and the requirement for distant medical care arrangements. Telehealth administrations offer people the accommodation of getting to medical services experts from the solace of their homes. Virtual wellbeing stages, then again, stretch out past conventional medical care to incorporate a wide exhibit of wellbeing administrations, from wellness classes and emotional well-being backing to sustenance directing.

The incorporation of telehealth and virtual health stages democratizes admittance to medical care and prosperity administrations, defeating geological hindrances and upgrading accommodation. Clients can participate in virtual discussions with medical care suppliers, take part in live-streamed wellness classes, and access customized health assets. The pattern towards virtualization mirrors a change in how people see and access medical services, underlining the significance of helpful and open wellbeing arrangements.

4. **Emotional wellness Tech and Stress The executives:**

Emotional well-being tech has arisen as an essential concentration inside the health tech scene, recognizing the natural association among mental and actual prosperity. Stress following and the board apparatuses, care applications, and virtual emotional wellness support administrations are acquiring unmistakable quality. Wearables furnished with biosensors can distinguish physiological markers of stress, inciting opportune mediations, for example, directed contemplation meetings or unwinding works out.

The rising commonness of emotional well-being tech mirrors a more extensive cultural acknowledgment of the significance of mental prosperity. People are looking for devices and assets that assist them with overseeing pressure, tension, and other psychological wellness challenges. This pattern lines up with a more comprehensive comprehension of health that goes past actual wellbeing to envelop mental and close to home viewpoints, underlining the interconnected idea of in general prosperity.

5. **Man-made reasoning for Customized Bits of knowledge:**

Man-made reasoning (artificial intelligence) assumes a focal part in the personalization of wellbeing arrangements, offering refined information examination and prescient capacities. Man-made intelligence calculations break down client information from wearables, wellbeing trackers, and different sources to recognize examples, connections, and potential wellbeing chances. These bits of knowledge empower the production of customized suggestions for nourishment, wellness, and generally prosperity.

For instance, man-made intelligence driven calculations can anticipate potential medical problems in light of changes in rest designs, action levels, and physiological boundaries. The combination of artificial intelligence with electronic wellbeing records (EHRs) further upgrades the capacity of medical services suppliers to offer customized care plans. The consistent learning nature of man-made intelligence guarantees that proposals advance with individual wellbeing directions, adding to proactive wellbeing the board.

6. **Biofeedback and Wearable Sensors:**

Biofeedback and wearable sensors address an arising pattern that enables people to screen and manage their physiological reactions effectively. Wearables outfitted with biofeedback sensors, for example, those estimating pulse inconstancy or skin conductance, give constant criticism on feelings of anxiety and close to home states. Clients can then take part in mediations, like profound breathing activities or directed reflection, to regulate their physiological reactions.

The joining of biofeedback into wearables adds to a more all encompassing way to deal with prosperity, perceiving the interconnectedness of physical and emotional wellness. These innovations give clients substantial input on the effect of pressure and way of life decisions on their physiological state, cultivating more noteworthy mindfulness and advancing proactive pressure the executives.

7. **Vivid Encounters and Health Applications:**

Vivid encounters and health applications are utilizing innovations like computer generated simulation (VR) and expanded reality (AR) to improve commitment and adequacy.

VR contemplation applications, for example, transport clients to peaceful conditions, encouraging unwinding and stress decrease. AR applications can overlay true conditions with data and prompts to help careful living.

The gamification of health encounters through vivid advances makes prosperity rehearses really captivating and pleasant. VR-based wellness exercises, for instance, give dynamic and intuitive work-out schedules that improve inspiration and adherence. The coordination of vivid encounters into wellbeing tech mirrors a developing accentuation on making wellbeing and prosperity exercises successful as well as pleasant and feasible.

8. **Nutrigenomics and Customized Nourishment:**

Nutrigenomics, the investigation of how individual hereditary varieties impact reactions to consume less calories, is building up some momentum in the wellbeing tech space. Progresses in hereditary testing and examination consider the recognizable proof of hereditary markers connected with supplement digestion, dietary inclinations, and awarenesses. This data is then used to tailor customized sustenance designs that line up with a person's hereditary inclinations.

Customized sustenance applications influence nutrigenomic experiences to suggest explicit dietary decisions in light of hereditary elements. For instance, people with an inclination to lactose narrow mindedness might get proposals for elective wellsprings of calcium. The mix of nutrigenomics into wellbeing tech mirrors a more profound comprehension of the interaction among hereditary qualities and way of life decisions, empowering more designated and powerful health intercessions.

9. **Blockchain for Information Security and Protection:**

As wellbeing tech depends progressively on the assortment and examination of touchy wellbeing information, guaranteeing the security and protection of this data is fundamental. Blockchain innovation is arising as a possible arrangement, giving a decentralized and secure system for overseeing wellbeing information. Blockchain permits people to have more noteworthy command over their wellbeing data, allowing consent for explicit substances to access and utilize their information while keeping up with protection and security.

Blockchain's alter safe nature improves the honesty of wellbeing records, forestalling unapproved adjustments. This decentralized methodology lines up with the standards of client driven command over private information, alleviating concerns connected with information breaks and unapproved access. Coordinating blockchain into wellbeing tech biological systems adds to building trust among clients, encouraging a solid and straightforward climate for wellbeing information the executives.

10. **Maintainability and Natural Wellbeing:**

A developing consciousness of natural manageability is impacting health tech patterns, with a rising accentuation on arrangements that advance both individual and ecological prosperity. Manageability centered health tech incorporates gadgets that screen ecological elements, like air quality and openness to contaminations. Also, health stages might integrate highlights that empower eco-accommodating ways of behaving, for example, maintainable sustenance decisions and carbon impression following.

The crossing point of wellbeing and maintainability mirrors a comprehensive comprehension of prosperity that reaches out past individual wellbeing to incorporate the strength of the planet. Clients are looking for health arrangements that line up with their upsides of natural stewardship, adding to a more extensive development towards eco-cognizant living.

**Difficulties and Contemplations:**

While the arising patterns and advances in wellbeing tech hold massive commitment, a few difficulties and contemplations should be tended to for far reaching reception and ideal effect. Protection concerns connected with the assortment and utilization of individual wellbeing information require vigorous shields. Executing straightforward information administration works on, getting educated assent, and guaranteeing consistence with security guidelines are fundamental stages in building and keeping up with client trust.

Interoperability stays a test as the health tech scene differentiates. Coordinating information from different gadgets, stages, and applications into strong wellbeing environments requires normalized information configurations and correspondence conventions. Cooperation among tech designers, medical services suppliers, and administrative bodies is significant in laying out interoperability norms that work with the consistent trade of data.

Moral contemplations encompassing computer based intelligence and AI calculations require cautious consideration. Guaranteeing decency, straightforwardness, and responsibility in algorithmic dynamic cycles is basic. Finding some kind of harmony between the advantages of artificial intelligence driven customized experiences and the moral utilization of information is fundamental for building client certainty and confidence in wellbeing tech arrangements.

**9.2 Discussion on the potential impact of quantum computing, nanotechnology, and other cutting-edge advancements**

The possible effect of state of the art progressions, for example, quantum figuring and nanotechnology on different areas, including medical services, materials science, and data innovation, is a subject of huge interest and investigation.

As these advancements keep on developing, their groundbreaking potential has the ability to reform the manner in which we approach complex issues and drive development in extraordinary ways.

1. **Quantum Registering:**

   Quantum registering addresses a change in perspective in computational capacities, utilizing the standards of quantum mechanics to perform calculations at speeds unfathomable with old style PCs. The likely effect on fields like medication revelation, advancement issues, and cryptography is significant.

   In drug revelation, for example, quantum PCs could mimic atomic cooperations with remarkable precision and speed. This could fundamentally assist the most common way of distinguishing new medications and figuring out their possible impacts on the human body. The capacity to reenact complex natural frameworks at the quantum level holds the commitment of opening novel restorative mediations and speeding up the advancement of medicines for different infections.

   Quantum registering likewise has suggestions for enhancement issues, where finding the best arrangement from countless conceivable outcomes is a computationally serious errand. Enterprises going from coordinated factors and store network the executives to fund and energy could profit from the quantum calculations that succeed at addressing advancement challenges. This might prompt more productive asset designation, cost decrease, and worked on by and large execution in different areas.

In the domain of cryptography, the approach of quantum processing brings the two difficulties and open doors. While it represents a danger to conventional cryptographic strategies, it likewise makes the way for quantum-safe cryptographic procedures. Scientists and enterprises are effectively dealing with creating quantum-safe calculations to guarantee the security of delicate data in the post-quantum period.

2. **Nanotechnology:**

Nanotechnology, the control of materials and gadgets at the nanoscale, holds tremendous commitment for various applications across assorted fields. In medical services, nanotechnology is ready to alter diagnostics, drug conveyance, and customized medication.

Symptomatic instruments at the nanoscale can recognize illnesses at a beginning phase with uncommon awareness. Nanoparticles designed to tie explicitly to biomarkers related with sicknesses empower early and precise conclusion. This early discovery ability can possibly altogether work on understanding results by taking into consideration opportune mediation and treatment.

Nanotechnology in drug conveyance includes the plan of nanoparticles that can move restorative specialists to explicit cells or tissues in the body. This designated drug conveyance limits aftereffects and upgrades the viability of medicines. Also, the capacity to design nanoparticles with properties, for example, supported discharge or set off discharge in light of explicit circumstances further extends the opportunities for redid restorative mediations.

In materials science, nanotechnology is making ready for the improvement of cutting edge materials with extraordinary properties. Nanomaterials display qualities like upgraded strength, conductivity, and reactivity because of their little size and expanded surface region. These materials track down applications in assembling, hardware, and environmentally friendly power, adding to the improvement of additional productive and manageable advances.

3. **Man-made consciousness (artificial intelligence) and AI (ML):**

The cooperative energy of quantum registering, nanotechnology, and man-made reasoning (computer based intelligence) is an especially convincing area of investigation. Quantum registering's capacity to handle huge measures of information in equal lines up with the information concentrated nature of computer based intelligence and AI calculations. Quantum AI calculations can possibly beat traditional partners in undertakings like example acknowledgment, enhancement, and complex information examination.

Nanotechnology, then again, can improve the equipment parts of man-made intelligence. The improvement of nanoscale gadgets and circuits can add to the production of all the more remarkable and energy-proficient processors. This could prompt huge headways in the speed and productivity of simulated intelligence applications, empowering the handling of enormous datasets continuously and working with more mind boggling computer based intelligence models.

The combination of these state of the art innovations could extraordinarily affect fields like medical services diagnostics and customized medication. For example, quantum AI calculations could investigate immense datasets of genomic data at remarkable velocities, prompting more exact and customized treatment suggestions in view of individual hereditary profiles.

4. **Data Security and Cryptography:**

The convergence of quantum figuring and cryptography is a region that requests cautious thought. While quantum figuring represents a danger to regular cryptographic strategies, it likewise presents a chance for the improvement of quantum-safe cryptographic procedures. Post-quantum cryptography is a functioning area of exploration zeroed in on making calculations that can endure the computational force of quantum PCs.

Nanotechnology can add to improving data security by giving new strategies to get correspondence and encryption. Nanoscale gadgets and materials could be used to foster imaginative cryptographic arrangements, guaranteeing the privacy and trustworthiness of computerized data despite developing innovative scenes.

5. **Ecological and Energy Applications:**

The likely effect of these headways stretches out past conventional areas to address squeezing worldwide difficulties, especially in the domains of energy and the climate. Quantum figuring and nanotechnology can assume significant parts in upgrading energy frameworks, materials plan for sustainable power advances, and the recreation of mind boggling ecological cycles.

Quantum PCs have the ability to show and mimic sub-atomic collaborations with high accuracy. This capacity is significant in planning new materials for effective energy stockpiling, catalysis, and sun based energy change. The capacity to computationally investigate and enhance materials at the quantum level could prompt leap forwards in the advancement of more feasible and energy-productive advances.

Nanotechnology adds to progressions in energy capacity, with nanomaterials offering expanded surface region and further developed conductivity for batteries and supercapacitors. Also, nanoscale sensors can be utilized to screen ecological circumstances and poisons, giving continuous information to more powerful natural administration.

**Difficulties and Contemplations:**

Regardless of the colossal capability of quantum processing, nanotechnology, and other state of the art headways, a few difficulties and contemplations should be addressed to understand their advantages completely.

1. **Specialized Difficulties:**
   Quantum PCs are right now in the beginning phases of advancement, with functional and adaptable quantum processing frameworks yet to be understood. Defeating specialized difficulties like blunder rectification, keeping up with quantum intelligence, and making stable qubits is urgent for the useful execution of quantum processing.
   Nanotechnology faces difficulties connected with adaptability and reproducibility. The blend and assembling of nanomaterials in enormous amounts with reliable properties present continuous difficulties. Guaranteeing the wellbeing and moral utilization of nanotechnology is another thought.

2. **Moral and Cultural Ramifications:**
   The quick headway of these advancements raises moral worries with respect to their expected abuse. Resolving issues connected with protection, security, and the mindful turn of events and sending of these advancements is principal.
   The cultural effect of occupation relocation because of computerization driven by simulated intelligence and AI is a worry. Setting up the labor force for the changing position scene and taking into account moral ramifications in computer based intelligence direction are basic angles that need consideration.

3. **Interdisciplinary Joint effort:**
   Effective coordination of quantum processing, nanotechnology, and simulated intelligence requires interdisciplinary joint effort among researchers, designers, policymakers, and ethicists. Overcoming any barrier between various disciplines is fundamental for comprehensive and dependable headways.
   Creating global guidelines and systems for the moral utilization of these advances is critical. A cooperative methodology will assist with tending to worldwide difficulties, for example, environmental change, medical services incongruities, and online protection dangers.

4. **Administrative Structures:**


Laying out administrative structures that guarantee the dependable turn of events and organization of these advancements is fundamental. Finding some kind of harmony between encouraging development and safeguarding people and social orders from potential dangers is a complex however important undertaking.

States, worldwide associations, and industry partners should cooperate to make administrative structures that address the worldwide idea of these advances while regarding different social and lawful settings.

**9.3 Ethical considerations and regulatory challenges in the future of health monitoring**

In the advancing scene of wellbeing observing advancements, moral contemplations and administrative difficulties are basic perspectives that request cautious consideration. As inventive arrangements keep on arising, guaranteeing the dependable turn of events, organization, and utilization of these advances becomes central for defending individual protection, advancing value, and keeping up with public trust.

Moral contemplations envelop a scope of issues, including the protection and security of individual wellbeing information. As wellbeing checking advancements gather progressively delicate data, it is significant to lay out vigorous shields to safeguard people from unapproved access and possible abuse of their information. Finding some kind of harmony between the advantages of information driven bits of knowledge and the insurance of individual protection requires straightforward information administration practices and client driven command over private wellbeing data.

Additionally, the evenhanded access and reasonableness of wellbeing observing innovations are moral objectives. Tending to differences in innovation access, computerized education, and medical services assets is fundamental to forestall the worsening of existing wellbeing imbalances. Moral structures ought to focus on inclusivity, guaranteeing that the advantages of cutting edge wellbeing checking are open to different populaces, independent of financial status or geological area.

Administrative difficulties in store for wellbeing observing rotate around the requirement for dynamic and versatile systems that can stay up with quickly advancing advancements. Policymakers should explore a complicated scene, taking into account the possible dangers and advantages of new developments while cultivating a climate helpful for advancement. Finding some kind of harmony between cultivating mechanical progressions and shielding general wellbeing is a sensitive undertaking that requires continuous cooperation between administrative bodies, industry partners, and medical services experts.

Normalizing administrative methodologies universally is another test, given the global idea of wellbeing checking advances. Creating firm structures that rise above geological limits requires cooperation among countries to guarantee predictable guidelines for information security, gadget wellbeing, and moral practices. Blending guidelines can upgrade interoperability, work with innovation reception, and lay out an underpinning of trust for clients and industry partners the same.

Moreover, moral contemplations stretch out to issues of straightforwardness and responsibility in algorithmic dynamic cycles. As man-made consciousness assumes an undeniably conspicuous part in wellbeing observing, guaranteeing reasonableness and alleviating predispositions in algorithmic results is basic. Laying out clear rules for the moral utilization of man-made intelligence in medical care, including wellbeing checking, is vital for construct and keep up with public trust.